T0224777

OPHTHALMOLOGISTS,

MEET ZERNIKE AND FOURIER!

Louis S. Jagerman, MD

©2007

Order this book online at www.trafford.com
or email orders@trafford.com

Most Trafford titles are also available at major online book retailers.

© Copyright 2008 Louis S. Jagerman MD.
All rights reserved. No part of this publication may be reproduced, stored in a retrieval system, or transmitted, in any form or by any means, electronic, mechanical, photocopying, recording, or otherwise, without the written prior permission of the author.

Print information available on the last page.

ISBN: 978-1-4251-3367-2 (sc)
ISBN: 978-1-4269-9049-6 (e)

Because of the dynamic nature of the Internet, any web addresses or links contained in this book may have changed since publication and may no longer be valid. The views expressed in this work are solely those of the author and do not necessarily reflect the views of the publisher, and the publisher hereby disclaims any responsibility for them.

Any people depicted in stock imagery provided by Getty Images are models, and such images are being used for illustrative purposes only.
Certain stock imagery © Getty Images.

Trafford rev. 07/13/2020

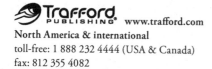 www.trafford.com

North America & international
toll-free: 1 888 232 4444 (USA & Canada)
fax: 812 355 4082

TABLE OF CONTENTS

ACKNOWLEDGMENTS

For their vital assistance in creating this book, I extend a special thanks to several individuals.

My associate and good friend Michael B. Limberg, MD[1] labored through my various manuscripts to help me write what I wished to convey.

Generous help was given by John A. Vukich, MD, Jack T. Holladay, MD, and Douglas D. Koch, MD.[2]

Proofreading was cheerfully provided by Ms. Lila Emmer,[3] who also guided me through my grammatical exploits.

The artwork and layout were expertly reworked by Randy Klemann.[4]

Of course my kind wife, Karen, patiently supported me through the lengthy and tedious process.

---

[1] San Luis Obispo, CA

[2] Madison, WI; Belaire, TX; and Houston, TX respectively.

[3] Bellingham, WA.

[4] D. B A. Graphics Northwest, Bellingham, WA.

INTRODUCTION

As if our profession were not complicated enough, we are now expected to know something about "Zernike polynomials," which reside in a branch of applied mathematics that plays a central role in contemporary refractive surgery. Moreover, recent developments have aroused interest in an alternative mathematical approach based on "Fourier polynomials," and the relative merits of these approaches are under scrutiny "as we speak."

My goal is to cover the nature and uses of Zernike and Fourier polynomials in sufficient detail so that my readers will know "what it's all about," particularly when mathematical terminology and nomenclature are used in discussing refractive surgery. In other words, I consider this form of mathematics to be another "basic science" which underpins contemporary ophthalmology, at least for refractive subspecialists. I also wish to prepare us for sophisticated patients who may otherwise know more than we do and whose concerns or questions may perplex us.

My qualifications stem from the practice of clinical ophthalmology for nearly 40 years, including some refractive surgery. I also studied mathematics in college, and I have previously published in this field; the list is on page 95.

The first section of this book covers two items, the mathematical side of preoperative measurements of refractive errors, and the ophthalmic uses of Zernike polynomials. The second section covers Fourier polynomials; it is shorter and somewhat less detailed because some material applies to both approaches. Nonetheless, the content of the second section is structured and footnoted so that readers familiar with Zernike may be satisfied by reading only the section on Fourier.

Since polynomials are not the only mathematical ingredients in these approaches, I use the terms "Zernike system" and "Fourier system" to identify the two main topics. I also use the plural terms "Zernike systems" and "Fourier systems" to emphasize that these systems exist in various forms, even though we will not explore all the nuances.

◆

In a wider perspective, refractive surgery consists of two main components. The first is the acquisition of the essential patient data, and this book is restricted to the mathematics behind the optical and refractive facets of this component. The second component is the execution of the surgery, notably with a laser, and I do not delve into this area, which primarily involves laser physics as well as the response of living tissues. Of course I must point out that the first component is more fundamental, in the same sense that underpins all of medicine: accurate diagnosis precedes successful therapy.

◆

For easy cross-referencing and efficient indexing of this complex topic, most paragraphs or groups of related paragraphs are numbered. My style is to write in the first person plural.

ZERNIKE POLYNOMIALS IN OPHTHALMOLOGY

A BIT OF HISTORY and the UNDERLYING PRINCIPLES

1.   Frits Zernike (1888-1966) was a Dutch physicist and mathematician deeply interested in optics. He won a Nobel prize for the invention of the phase-contrast microscope, but in the process he devised a method for the analysis of optical aberrations. The latter was initially applied to optical instruments, notably telescopes. That is to say, Zernike polynomials were not designed for ophthalmologists but for astronomers and optical engineers. Therefore, when panels of experts (see Note 1 on page 89) selected Zernike polynomials as the preferred mathematical system for refractive surgery less than 10 years ago, they were advocating a novel use for a pre-existing mathematical tool. However, the choice is very logical, since many of the optical defects that plague telescopes are very similar to those that commonly afflict human eyes. Indeed the Zernike approach serves us quite well, though we will discuss some of its drawbacks.

2.   The application we are looking at is in the realm of "adaptive optics." A good example of adaptive optics is the auto-focus camera. A device in the camera senses when it is not in focus, and this information is used to "adapt" the optics automatically. In effect, the camera performs refractive surgery on itself. We can even think of ocular accommodation as an innate form of adaptive optics.

3.   A stimulus to the development of adaptive optics came from the "Star Wars" program in the 1980's, in which weapons are guided by optical devices that must allow error-free imaging of targets. As is also true in astronomy, the main source of aberrations in this setting is atmospheric turbulence, but systems have been designed to monitor the aberrations and compensate for them instantly. The compensation is usually achieved by way of flexible "deformable" mirrors.

4.   An intermediate stage in the evolution of adaptive optics was reached in Germany in the early 1990's when scanning laser ophthalmoscopy was modified for improved retinal tomography. (The name associated with this key development is J. Liang. See Bibliography.) The first commercial adaptive-optics devices for PRK and LASIK were built in the late 1990's. We can therefore think of refractive surgery as leisurely ophthalmic adaptive optics, in which we compensate for refractive errors by altering—"deforming"—the eye. Of course we rely on the fact that the cornea is eminently "deformable."

5.   It appears we can even go further with adaptive optics on humans. If we remove all ocular optical aberrations, we may create "supernormal" vision, limited only by the resolving power of foveal cones. Indeed, full elimination of aberrations may allow better than 20/10 visual acuity, and treated patients may justifiably claim that they "have never seen this well."

◆

6.   A major problem for clinical ophthalmology is the plethora of synonyms used for the technical and mathematical entities that play a role in the optical aspects of refractive surgery. Moreover, despite efforts to standardize the terminology, diverse methods and customs are accepted in the organization of the material, and significant disagreements exist on some conventions, mathematical steps, and systems of equations.

7. Nonetheless, the underlying principle is familiar. An emmetropic eye will accurately focus parallel rays of light on its retina, and an ametropic eye will fail to do so. (To be precise, we do not deal with rays of light, only small bundles of rays, but we can ignore this detail. Such bundles may be called "beamlets.") We also use the principle that the optical behavior of emitted light is identical to that of entering light.[5] As in manual retinoscopy, we can illuminate the posterior retina with light and then gauge the parallel-ness of reflected and emitted rays. An appropriate light source for retinal illumination is a HeNe laser. Such light, upon reflection off the retina, exits the eye through the pupil, and all refractive errors affect the rays passing through the pupil. (Any light that leaves the eye appears to come out at the "exit pupil.") The emitted light has a "*wavefront*," which is a cardinal ingredient in Zernike as well as in Fourier systems.

8. To envision a wavefront, we imagine that all the emitted light forms a beam which has the diameter of the pupil, and that we can examine the face of this beam in or near the pupillary plane. This face is the wavefront; think of looking at the end of a pencil eraser. Of course we cannot "see" the wavefront itself; it is a theoretical structure made of photons caught in a moment of time as they exit the eye. Nevertheless, we can determine the theoretical shape of the wavefront. Once this shape has been ascertained, we create pictures, maps, and topographic models of it, and of course the ultimate use of this information is to remedy the deformities in that shape surgically.

9. The key concept here is that *we can determine the shape of the wavefront by examining the parallel-ness of the emitted rays of light.* When all rays exiting the eye are parallel, the wavefront is presumed to be perfectly flat, and when the eye has aberrations—when the rays exiting the eye are not all parallel—the wavefront is presumed not to be flat. (See Note 2 on page 89.) From the shape of the wavefront we identify and quantify the optical aberrations of the eye. Therefore, *the shape of the wavefront is treated as a complete representation of the refractive state of the eye.* The requisite for refractive surgery then is "know thy wavefront," and Zernike systems treat wavefronts as shapes. Ergo, "know thy shape."

10. To gauge the behavior of exiting rays for their parallel-ness, they are focused as "spots" on a reference plane. Light sensors built into this reference plane gather the necessary information, and the exact locations of the spots are the critical data. The brightest points of these spots are "centroids," and using centroids to gauge the wavefront is called the "centroid method." We will describe the typical method, equipment, and technical problems in detail.

11. When the wavefront deviates from flatness because of ametropia, we can say that a "wavefront error" exists, commonly abbreviated as a "WFE." Therefore, *a wavefront error at some point on the wavefront is a gap between where the wavefront surface would have been without aberrations and where it is in the presence of aberrations.* Think of two very thin pieces of plywood, one of which is as flat as it should be, and another which is warped. When the two surfaces are brought together so they just touch, gaps between them will exist. In this sense, we simply measure wavefront errors—gaps—at many locations. "Aberrometry" is the process of measuring wavefront errors, though in effect it is a specialized kind of refraction, particularly in the context of refractive surgery. (A synonym for aberrometry which occasionally reaches ophthalmic literature is "metrology.")

---

[5] In theoretical physics this is not absolutely accurate.

12. An important consequence of the absence of all aberration is that the wavefront has no slope. Of course this is the same as saying that it is flat and that no aforementioned gaps (no WFE's) exist. However, some critical mathematics—which we will examine—hinges on the fact that *in the presence of aberrations the wavefront surface will have a slope at some or all locations.* We therefore say that the perfectly flat wavefront has "zero slope everywhere," and this is a very useful notion.

Despite a subtle technical distinction, a "slope" is often referred to as a "gradient." We will therefore hear that an "aberrated" wavefront has gradients at one or more—usually at many—locations. "Aberrated" means from an eye with any refractive error. Looking ahead, knowing the slopes or gradients at enough locations allows us to calculate the shape of the wavefront.

13. Not every defect of an optical system is effectively addressed in this manner. Just as contemporary LASIK does not eradicate chromatic aberration, scattering, and certain kinds of light-wave diffraction, likewise these processes do not enter into the usual analysis of the wavefront. Indeed this still is one of the limitations of Zernike's system in improving the design of optical equipment in general.

14. Incidentally, not all systems for aberrometry require that the retina reflect and emit light. The Tscherning aberrometer places fine spots in a certain regular pattern on the posterior retina. The pattern is photographed and analyzed for changes away from the expected regularity. A similar system is attributed to the ideas of Scheiner (who was a surprisingly sophisticated pioneer in physiologic optics 400 years ago).

15. We may also encounter the concept that, in the absence of aberrations, all rays entering through the pupil of the eye are "in phase" with each other (in step with each other with respect to waves of light) when they reach the macula. Then, "phase defects" represent refractive errors. We need not elaborate on this approach, but two corollaries are noteworthy.

First, as a theoretical concept, any wavefront (with or without aberrations) is said to be a surface of constant phase. That is to say, all rays that reflect off the retina and form the surface of the wavefront (whether it is flat or not) are in phase with each other. Each ray has undergone the same number of wave cycles while passing through the ocular media, even if that media retarded some rays and not others.

Second, it is possible to describe the refractive status of the eye mathematically in terms of phase. Clinical literature rarely uses such descriptions, but research articles may do so. Therefore, we need not elaborate on this concept but should be aware of it.

HARTMANN-SHACK in the ZERNIKE SYSTEM

16. The standard instrument for determining the shape of wavefront is the "Hartmann-Shack wavefront sensor," or "H-S aberrometer," or simply "H-S device," though it is sometimes called the Shack-Hartmann device. Hartmann, a German astrophysicist, designed this device to identify a flaw in a large telescope about a century ago. Shack later added the lenslets to Hartmann's device; we will describe these shortly. For brevity we henceforth use the initials H-S for Hartmann-Shack. Besides H-S devices, other instruments have been designed for this purpose, but we will not detail these.

17. The immediate task of a H-S device is to *deduce the shape of the wavefront*. This requires a small flat screen placed some distance away from the exit pupil, as if for projecting slides. That distance must be long enough to tell whether a thin ray precisely illuminates a preselected location on the screen. We call this screen our "reference plane," which we already mentioned in paragraph 10 and which we will describe in detail later.

18. One important refinement (devised by Shack) is an array of very small convex lenses inserted just after the exit pupil so as to focus each ray onto the reference plane. Such a lens is a "lenslet," and each lenslet must be accurately embedded into an opaque screen; a diagram appears on page 13. This arrangement creates a grid of bright spots of light on the reference plane which are sufficiently discreet so that their exact locations (the location of each centroid, to be precise) are evident. As we will describe later, lenslets allow modern H-S aberrometers to use very small video sensors in the reference plane to detect—"capture"—the spots.

◆

19. Since locations on the reference plane are critical in this approach, we need a detour to discuss several details about the identification of locations in the H-S sensor. Two methods for marking locations are with *Cartesian coordinates* and with *spherical polar coordinates*. The former is the familiar two-dimensional x-y system, where x is the horizontal coordinate or axis, and y is vertical. This method is intuitively simple, particularly for identifying locations on the reference plane. A location is given by a pair of numbers, often written as "(x, y)."

(A word of warning: some conventions reverse x and y axes, which can lead to confusion when sources are compared. Others routinely include the third dimension, z, which is largely superfluous for our discussions.)

20. However, for many purposes an alternative is preferred, the spherical polar system, which lends itself better to trigonometric analysis, especially on circular surfaces. The coordinates of a two-dimensional spherical polar system are a *radius* measured from the center of the surface, and an *angle* measured from a reference meridian. Hence a spherical polar system is also called a radial system. In our instance, the radius is given by ρ , and the meridional angle by θ. A location is given by a pair of numbers, often written as "(ρ, θ)."

21. Diagrams of these systems of coordinates follow on the next page.

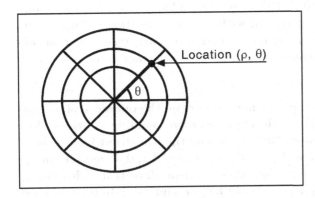

A typical two-dimensional spherical polar system of coordinates.

A location is identified by two numbers. One is a radius (ρ) and the other is an angle (θ).

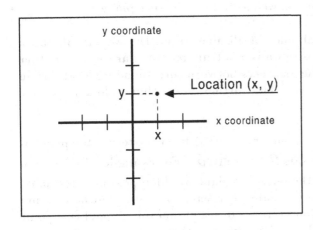

A typical two-dimensional Cartesian system of coordinates.

A location is identified by two numbers, x and y.

22. A spherical polar system lends itself well to identifying locations on the circular surface of a wavefront. For this purpose we customarily consider the maximum radius of that surface to have a numerical value of 1 (one). A wavefront—and hence the pupil—become "unit circles." This is accomplished by the equation $\rho = r / a$, where a is the radius of the exit pupil of the eye and r is the distance from a spot to the center. If $r = a$, then $\rho = 1$. The range for ρ is therefore zero to 1. We say that ρ is the "normalized" radial distance in the unit circle. (More on normalization later.)

This means that Zernike polynomials are defined in a circular pupil which always has a unit radius—a radius of 1—no matter what its real size. (The mathematical definition of a polynomial is not essential for us at this point; it will be covered in paragraph 52.) If we wish to assign a real size to the wavefront to match the pupil, each ρ is multiplied by the pupil radius. Thus if the pupil radius is 3 mm, a location with a ρ of 0.5 is 1.5 mm from the center. We will see that the fundamental equation of Zernike's system, presented in paragraph 136, is best solved on a unit circle. This in turn means that under many circumstances, but not all, spherical polar systems are "natural" for Zernike's mathematics. Nevertheless, let us set this concept aside for later use, as for now we can rely on the simpler Cartesian coordinates.

23.   For convenience we superimpose an *x-y* Cartesian set of coordinates on the reference plane as well as on the wavefront. We ensure that every location on the reference plane, as identified by a unique value for *x* and for *y,* is directly across from a location on the wavefront that has the same *x* and *y*. The lenslets are also aligned with the same locations. This means that *if the emitted rays are all parallel—if the wavefront is truly flat—then every point on this wavefront must lie directly in line with every corresponding point on a reference plane*. We see a diagram of this on page 13.

24.   Under these conditions—namely emmetropia—video sensors on the reference plane will detect the spots of light from the lenslets exactly at the expected corresponding locations. For example, let us consider the beam emanating from the location on the wavefront labeled as "$x = 0.2$ and $y = 0.3$" (or simply "0.2, 0.3"); it will pass through the "0.2, 0.3" lenslet, and it will strike the reference plane at the "0.2, 0.3" location, where a sensor detects it. This means that every ray emanating from the emmetropic eye should be perpendicular to (in technical language, should be "normal to") the wavefront as well as to the reference plane.

25.   It is also useful to visualize that in absence of all aberration, the wavefront and a reference plane are precisely parallel, like opposite walls of a truly rectangular room. In other words, when there are no wavefront errors, the distances between corresponding locations on the wavefront and reference plane are all the same. This further means that all locations show zero slope.

26.   Incidentally, it is possible to transform (convert, switch) from Cartesian to spherical polar coordinates by use of the equations $x = r\cos\theta$, $y = r\sin\theta$. For example, the location "$x = 0.2, y = 0.3$" in Cartesian coordinates on the reference plane would appear as "$\rho = 0.36$, $\theta = 56°$" in polar coordinates. Using these coordinates, it is easy to ensure that no location falls outside a space with a maximum dimension of $\rho = 1.0$; see paragraph 22, and this point will resurface when we get to place Zernike polynomials into equations.

27.   This is an opportunity for a comment on an idiosyncrasy in how these two systems of coordinates are applied in ophthalmology. When we face a patient, for both eyes the angle θ is set up to be zero at the 3 o'clock meridian and to rotate counterclockwise. Likewise, when an *x-y* system is used, for both eyes, *x* is positive going to our right and negative going to our left. (We say that these are "right-handed" systems for OU.) Because of this custom, certain quantities which are positive for one eye turn out to be negative for the other. Also, at times a "*z*" coordinate is included which runs along the line of sight, but as testing is done on light reflected from the retina, *z* is set up positive advancing out of the eye. Ergo, some values again turn out to be unexpectedly negative. Fortunately, a conversion has been agreed upon which resolves any right-left discrepancies; what is positive for OD is positive for OS, etc.

28.   In summary, *in the absence of all aberrations,* several criteria are met (and we use the term "everywhere" for "all locations"): (1) All rays are parallel "everywhere" in the pupil. (2) All rays are perpendicular "everywhere." (3) The wavefront has zero slope "everywhere." (4) The wavefront and reference plane are equidistant "everywhere," and if they were brought together, no gaps would exist between them. (5) Each ray passes through the aligned corresponding locations on the wavefront, through the lenslet, and onto the reference plane. (6) All video sensors detect rays—in the form of focused spots (centroids)—directly in line with the optical center of each lenslet at the corresponding expected locations on the reference plane.

29. From the point of view of methodology, the last of these criteria is the most important, because what H-S sensors "sense" is the location of each spot of light (centroid) when the ray reaches the reference plane. Thus if the emitted rays are *not* parallel—if the wavefront is not flat everywhere and has a slope anywhere—*then some or all spots of light will show a displacement.* The spots will not end up at their expected or anticipated locations. Of course this means that the eye has optical aberrations; it has refractive errors. As we will see in detail later, *aberrations are identified and measured by the patterns of displacements of spots of light on the reference plane.*

30. This arrangement, whereby data gathered on the two-dimensional reference plane is used to generate a picture of the three-dimensional wavefront, demonstrates a profound mathematical concept: Two-dimensional data, such as x's and y's or ρ's and θ's, suffices to reveal the three-dimensional shape of the wavefront. Why is that significant? Because surgery is three-dimensional.

31. Just as is true for the locations of the spots, their displacements on the reference plane can be expressed in Cartesian or in spherical polar coordinates. However, Cartesian coordinates are easier to use here, since the spots are usually projected by the lenslets onto the reference plane as a square grid with straight rows and columns like a chess board. *Then a side-to-side displacement of any spot (any centroid, to be precise) can be labeled as Δx and an up-and-down displacement as Δy.* (Yes, corners of this lattice are cut since it is a square placed into a basically circular system. This detail represents a technical problem.)

◆

32. In paragraph 12 we introduced the notion that an aberrated wavefront—one which is affected by refractive errors—has slopes (gradients) at various x-y locations. To appreciate the technologic details in a typical H-S device as it is used in a Zernike system, we should examine more closely how the Δx and Δy displacements are linked to the determination of slopes.

33. Each location on the reference plane holds a cluster of very small closely spaced CCD video sensors (CCD's or coupled change devices, a.k.a. "detector pixels") which can detect the level of illumination that reaches them. Usually a cluster consists of a square of 4 or 9 pixels. These clusters of sensors are called subapertures, with each subaperture assigned to one lenslet and one specific location. In the absence of aberrations, the center of each spot—the centroid—falls into the very center of its corresponding subaperture. In the presence of aberrations, one spot may activate several sensors unevenly within each subaperture. A computerized algorithm pools data from individual sensors; just how comes later. We note that in effect the lenslets subdivide the light from the wavefront into a collection of rays, and by studying the locations of these rays—i.e., the locations of the spots—on the video sensors, we will be able to "reconstruct" the wavefront.

34. The diagram on page 13 depicts a simplified system. Light from a wavefront (upper left corner) reaches a screen with 16 lenslets. These lenslets are labeled with Cartesian coordinates **x, y**. We consider only the ray that passes through lenslet $x_4\,y_3$. This ray reaches subaperture $x_4\,y_3$ on the reference plane. The lower part of the diagram shows this aperture in detail. In this case the spot (the circle) and centroid (the dot) for this ray are displaced; there exists a Δx towards the right and a smaller Δy upwardly.

We recall (paragraph 18) that each spot on the reference plane has a certain brightness to it, maximum at its centroid. Arrays of sensors (pixels) detect the locations of brightest illumination. For instance, pixel sensor "I" and "II" should receive equal brightness when the wavefront is flat, and yet here sensor "II" to the right of sensor "I" detects more brightness. The system then "knows" that an aberration exists which created a displacement and hence a slope to the right at this location. The difference in brightness quantifies this local slope. The aim of this process is to assemble local slopes at many positions across the pupil.

In the diagram, the subaperture contains four pixel sensors labeled I, II, III and IV. As we said, these sensors record the amount of illumination each receives. The ray forms a spot which has a centroid that falls inside pixel II. The ray also partly illuminates pixels I, III and IV. Let us assume the following:

Pixel I senses 0.2 relative intensity of illumination.
Pixel II senses 0.6 relative intensity of illumination.
Pixel III senses 0.1 relative intensity of illumination.
Pixel IV senses 0.3 relative intensity of illumination.

If there were no displacement at this location, all four pixels would "capture" the same intensity. They would be equally illuminated.

Using the above data, slope (gradient) of illumination in x-direction is proportional to

$$\frac{(II+IV)-(I+III)}{I+II+III+IV}=0.5.$$

The slope of illumination in y-direction is proportional to

$$\frac{(III+IV)-(I+II)}{I+II+III+IV}=-0.33$$

which is this case is negative because in the diagram down is positive.

In summary, the slope of wavefront at location x_4 y_3 is 0.5 in x-direction (to the right) and 0.33 in y-direction (downwardly). These are the crucial data.

35. If the displacements are so large or the subaperture so small that a spot from one lenslet illuminates another's subaperture, the algorithm may be "fooled" into reporting a spurious result. Think of an inept archer in a tournament whose arrow hits the neighboring archer's target. The requirement for an acceptable size of subapertures limits the number of spots and subapertures on a technical basis. Each spot must also be clear and well focused. These considerations, and others we will cite, contribute to limiting the number of usable spots to about 40, even though a modern H-S device can accommodate at least 240 spots or lenslets. Once we discuss the Fourier system, this number, 40, will be important, though the pupil size is critical. (For simplicity we included only 16 spots in the diagram.)

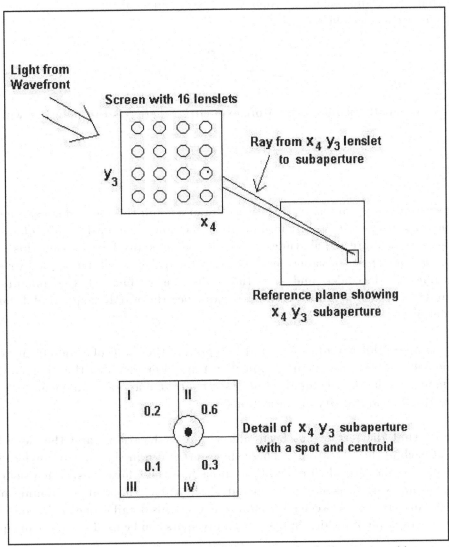

A diagram of a simplified H-S device. Please see text beginning on page 11.

36.   The associated mathematics proceeds as follows: We need to express slopes as angles. Accordingly we can call the local slope—i.e., the average slope or gradient at any location marked by x, y—angle S. As before, we label the displacement of the spots by Δx's and Δy's, since Cartesian coordinates work well here. The distance from the lenslets to the focal plane is f, which is their focal distance. From basic trigonometry, any Δ in the x or y direction is such that

$$\Delta = f\,\frac{S}{\sqrt{1+S^2}}$$

but because the slope is slight compared to f (the human wavefront is not extremely jagged), the denominator is practically 1 (one).

This means that each displacement is proportional to the angle of the local slope, so that in our context the adequate equation is

$$\Delta = f\,\frac{S}{1}$$

The 1 in the denominator is unneeded. More explicitly, where S is the angle, we will use

$$\frac{\Delta(x\,or\,y)}{f} = S$$

37.   Here we apply a useful analogy, the creation of a small three-dimensional model of the wavefront in a manner in which we could create a map and then a 3-D model of a mountain. The data for this task are the altitudes or elevations at many locations on this mountain. Locations are given as pairs of values for x and y (in Cartesian coordinates), and we can think of these values as latitudes and longitudes on the surface of the mountain. (The latitude/longitude system is not exactly Cartesian since the Earth is spheroidal, but we can ignore this detail.)

Of course the shape of this mountain is meant to represent the shape of a wavefront, while such maps and models are very useful in a clinical setting. For instance the "jaggedness" of a wavefront model or the density of the lines in a contour map of a wavefront is a graphic reflections of the clinical severity of aberrations.

Let us assume that the terrain has been sampled at 40 locations, and the slope has been determined at each of these locations. These slopes are given in the form of angles. Our task requires calculating the altitude (or elevation) at each of these locations. Each such location is said to be "local," since it is only one element of the entire shape of the mountain, but the process entails comparisons between adjacent elements. This detail is one of the considerations (mentioned in paragraph 35) which limits how many spots can be used this type of equipment.

Converting the angles to altitudes will not be difficult. The key will be that a slope at some location is a change in the altitude at that location. This inference is more obvious if we consider, say, three locations in a row, each of which has a steeper slope and hence a greater angle; clearly, the altitude is increasing from one spot to the next. Then (once we agree on a scale) by assembling these altitudes at their respective locations, the "reconstruction" of contour maps and three-dimensional models of the mountain poses no problems.

This analogy is meant to elicit how the wavefront—its shape, to be more precise—is reconstructed from the raw data provided usually by a H-S device. As we detailed, these data arise from displacements of spots that are converted to a collection of slopes.

Another feature of the analogy is a reference altitude which we can think of as sea level (as long as we acknowledge that some of the terrain can be "below sea level" because, as we shall see later, the wavefront can have valleys as well as peaks). This means that we can attach a meaningful numerical value to each altitude (again assuming we agree on a scale). In the case of a mountain, these values might be feet or meters, but what our model depicts is so small that microns are appropriate.

38. Let us recall the concept of the *wavefront error* (paragraph 11). By that definition, an error at some point on the wavefront is a gap between where the wavefront surface would have been without aberrations and where it is in the presence of aberrations. Instead of envisioning wavefront errors as gaps between two sheets of plywood, our mountain analogy treats these errors as gaps between a "sea level" and each of the 40 locations on our mountain. Of course these gaps are our "altitudes."

The next section deals with some mathematical details about wavefront errors.

The WAVEFRONT ABERRATION FUNCTION

39. At this juncture we introduce a very important mathematical term, the *wavefront aberration function*, also called the *wavefront error function*. In spherical polar coordinates it is labeled as

$$W(\rho, \theta)$$

but since Cartesian coordinates are easier to work with at the moment, our wavefront aberration function is labeled as

$$W(x, y) \, .$$

This deceptively simple term stands for the entire collection of wavefront errors (WFE's). In this case we assume that it is a set of "altitudes" at 40 locations (in other terms, 40 "gaps"), which means that it represents *the shape of the wavefront*! As we will detail, this mathematical entity quantifies *the total optical status of this eye*.

The efficiency of $W(x, y)$ is clearer if we realize that it stands for a collection of numbers assigned to each location, and therefore each location is linked to a value of x and y. In the above diagram we focused on one location, where $x = 4$ and $y = 3$. If we wished to write out all elements for a typical case, $W(x, y)$ could contain 80 numbers, corresponding to 40 x-y pairs. Thus $W(x, y)$ is really a mathematical repository of information which enables us to delineate the shape of the entire wavefront in a compact manner.

40. Many authors use "optical path differences" rather than wavefront errors to describe wavefronts. The "altitude" in the wave aberration function is analogous to the optical path difference (OPD) between the length of a ray at some point on the wavefront and the length of an unaberrated ray. Both the WFE and the OPD therefore represent a distance between the wavefront surface and the reference plane at some location, and both can be expressed in microns, but by convention they have opposite algebraic signs. (The $+$ or $-$ depends on whether the z-direction of the rays emitted out of the eye during aberrometry is considered positive or negative.) Renditions of wavefronts which are convex based on OPD turn out to be concave based on WFE, and vice versa. To inter-convert these quantities, OPD $= -$ WFE; in effect, OPD's are negative altitudes, i.e., depths.

41. Common sense alone dictates that if data from more points can be assembled, our wavefront aberration function will have greater fidelity. However, it turns out that a huge amount is neither technically feasible, nor is it always desirable. But in any case, the process for delineating the wavefront aberration function—i.e., for obtaining the shape of the wavefront from that data—is called *reconstruction*, because the wavefront in effect is first broken up by the lenslets into local elements and then it is reassembled. We will now examine this important process in some detail.

42.   Relying on Cartesian equations, we apply the notion that each component of $W(x, y)$ is like an altitude as well as a wavefront error. Hence the slope of the altitude in the x-direction is

$$\frac{\partial W(x,y)}{\partial x}$$

and in the y-direction it is

$$\frac{\partial W(x,y)}{\partial y}.$$

These two terms are examples of partial differentials or partial derivatives. A differential, a.k.a. a derivative, calculates the change in a quantity. (Acceleration is a differential of speed.) To perform differentiation, a quantity is mathematically partitioned into very small segments. When more than one quantity changes independently, the differentials are partial. Here two quantities change, simply because our measurements were made in two independent dimensions, x and y.

Next we apply the conclusion (from paragraph 36) that the angles of the local slopes can be calculated from the displacements according to

$$\frac{\Delta(x \, or \, y)}{f} = S.$$

43.   Therefore we can link slopes with displacements, such that

$$\frac{\partial W(x,y)}{\partial x} = \frac{\Delta x}{f} \quad and \quad \frac{\partial W(x,y)}{\partial y} = \frac{\Delta y}{f}.$$

The assembly of all slopes is then represented by $W(x, y)$, and it describes the shape of the wavefront built from the calculated wavefront errors, each of which is the deviation from flatness at some location. In short, during reconstruction of the wavefront we have progressed as follows:

Displacements of spots → Slopes → Wavefront errors → Shape of wavefront,

and the corresponding symbols are

$$\Delta x\text{'s and } \Delta y\text{'s} \rightarrow S\text{'s} \rightarrow W\text{'s} \rightarrow W(x, y).$$

Of course the shape of the wavefront in this form is only a list of wavefront errors. The problem, to be addressed soon, is to identify the refractive errors which are contained in the wavefront.

44. The mathematical method for pooling data in order to generate a map or model involves "integration," as in "integral calculus," which is like reassembling something that had been partitioned into very small segments. We say that the local altitudes—or more precisely the local slopes, one for each location—are "integrated over the subaperture" and "over the reference plane" to create the three-dimensional wavefront. In a sense, integration is the opposite of differentiation; the former adds together what the latter has disassembled.

We will revisit integration because it is used somewhat differently in Fourier systems, and this difference has clinical implications.

45. So far we ignored what each "altitude" really represents in analytic terms. Suppose that an eye has 14 Zernike polynomials contained in its total refractive error, each of which stems from a different aberration, which is not at all peculiar (since an eye can have that many aberrations). In other words, the optical status is described by these 14 polynomials. This means that every single "altitude" on the wavefront—earlier we envisioned 40 altitudes—reflects an algebraic compilation of 14 other pieces of information. In more technical language, the numerical value of each locus on the wavefront is the resultant of 14 underlying values.

The mountain analogy is weak on this facet, as we would have to imagine 14 different "geologic" forces or factors coming together to determine the altitude at each location. However, based on clinical experience we can imagine a simpler instance, such as a case with only two elementary aberrations, say myopia and astigmatism. This eye most likely has two or three Zernike polynomials represented in its total refractive error, which means that every "altitude" on the wavefront reflects an algebraic compilation of two or three other pieces of information. This concept impels us finally to call upon individual Zernike polynomials as well their sums, as we shall do in the next sections.

There is a reason for the words "most likely" in the previous paragraph. Later we will see how polynomials can describe myopia and astigmatism in a Zernike system, but often this is not so simple. For instance, depending on the axis, one polynomial may not suffice to describe just astigmatism, and indeed many aberrations require more than one polynomial for their mathematical description.

ZERNIKE POLYNOMIALS

46.   Since the Zernike polynomial is the protagonist, let us now define it in detail. Each Zernike polynomial is a mathematical description of an optical aberration or at times merely one feature of a complex aberration. For economy of words let us say that *Zernike polynomials depict aberrations*. Thus if we have detected "myopia with astigmatism," we can say that we have detected—as a preview of a Zernike polynomial—"$\rho^2 \cos 2\theta$ ".

Incidentally, other rarely used mathematical systems can do the same. For example Seidel polynomials are available to depict aberrations. However, unlike Zernike's polynomials, Seidel's were designed for industrial optics, and they have some mathematical disadvantages. The main issue is that they are not independent of each other (not "orthogonal" in geometric terms), which means that they are not as reliable for clinical use to treat complicated (high-order) aberrations.

47.   It is important that the description "$\rho^2 \cos 2\theta$ " only *identifies* the kind of aberration; it does not quantify it. The *amount* of myopia and astigmatism will require another number to go along with "$\rho^2 \cos 2\theta$." That is to say, unlike an "Rx" which tells us both the kind of aberration and its magnitude, a Zernike polynomial alone only relates the former. As we will see, the number which expresses the magnitude or amount of an aberration gives each Zernike polynomial a "weight."

48.   Another way of thinking about Zernike polynomials is that each one represents one pre-defined particular shape which may be found in a wavefront. For instance the Zernike polynomial for myopia describes a wavefront which has a concavity, and Zernike polynomials for myopia-and-astigmatism combinations describe wavefronts with a warped concavity.

Incidentally, the hyperopic eye has a convex wavefront; emitted rays reflected from the retina diverge unless re-converged by a convex corrective lens. Myopia and hyperopia are called "defocus" or (rarely) "power," while "astigmatism" is called just that in the Zernike system.

49.   We will see (e.g., paragraph 93) that an individual Zernike polynomial only describes one kind of aberration, or at the most, one feature of one "family." It does not cover many possibilities together, and when it deals with more than one defect—e.g., defocus and astigmatism, trefoil and coma—it is because these are cooperatively interrelated. Thus no single polynomial handles astigmatism *and* spherical aberration *and* coma. On the other hand we can add different Zernike polynomials together to obtain a comprehensive representation of the overall aberration of an eye. The complexities of how polynomials cooperate are discussed in paragraphs 180-189. In any case, the list of polynomials which goes into the overall aberration becomes a comprehensive description of that aberration. As we will see, such a list forms a "weighted sum" of polynomials, since each polynomial is given a "weight."

50.   The natural question here is why bother with apparently cumbersome Zernike polynomials. The answer is that a H-S device—or any other aberrometer—only supplies raw mathematical data about the wavefront, requiring that we break its shape down into more manageable ingredients. *These "ingredients" are the Zernike polynomials*, and the process of breaking down the wavefront into Zernike polynomials is best called "*analysis*," though some name it "decomposition," as is sometimes more intuitive.

Through analysis, the Zernike polynomials enable us to express the complex raw data as clinically meaningful descriptions of the patient's optical status, which can then be used to remedy the errors. In the case of LASIK, this entails wavefront-guided ablation (See Note 3 on page 89) with an excimer laser, applying bursts of intense ultraviolet light to sever bonds between corneal collagen molecules. As we said, this process is the ophthalmologic equivalent of adaptive optics.

51.   Incidentally, the ground-breaking equation that tells us how much ablation of the cornea is needed to induce one diopter's worth of flattening of the wavefront is called the Munnerlyn Formula, named for one of the pioneers of excimer laser ablation in refractive surgery.

Another incidental issue is whether measurements of aberrations are stable through time. Indeed we know that the refractive status fluctuates quickly—it a matter of seconds—even without natural accommodation. Meanwhile Zernike polynomials tacitly presume that refractive errors are stable. However, this is not a major impediment in clinical practice.

$$\blacklozenge$$

52.   If a Zernike polynomial is a mathematical identification of an optical aberration, why is it a polynomial? The full technical definition of a polynomial is not critical for us, but in essence it is an algebraic sum of several mathematical terms which have a constant and a variable raised to a positive integer power (an exponent). The quantity x^2+3x-4 is a typical polynomial, but some of these terms can be zero, and the power (exponent) can be 1 and therefore may not be written out.

Though every Zernike polynomial has a polynomial part, we will see that not every part is a polynomial. E.g., not every part of "$\rho^2 \cos 2\theta$" is a polynomial. Ergo "Zernike polynomial" is somewhat of a misnomer. A more accurate term for Zernike polynomials is "Zernike polynomial products," though it is rarely used, but it is based on the idea that a true polynomial is one of their factors.

53.   We will find several synonyms for "Zernike polynomial(s)." Frequently encountered refractive errors, such as tilt, coma, astigmatism, spherical aberration, defocus (myopia and hyperopia), etc., are called "modes" in the context of Zernike's mathematics. (In another sense, the Zernike system is a "modal" approach as opposed to a zonal approach; this detail is not essential for us.) Therefore, we routinely use the word "mode" as an alternative to Zernike polynomial. Another synonym is "aberration," which is rather general, but we also use this term for a Zernike polynomial.

54.   A further mathematically cogent alternative is "Zernike basis function." The rationale for "basis" is that individual Zernike polynomials can be added to form a weighted sum, which makes each Zernike polynomial a "basis" for that sum. (This term stems from vector algebra. A member of a sum is also called an "addend.") As for the term "function," in this setting its simple definition is some *numerical relationship between mathematical variables*; "myopia is a function of axial length." A working definition of a function is anything expressible by an equation. Calling Zernike polynomials "functions" is quite rational, for they indeed are mathematical relationships, as we will see.

Two additional definitions are pertinent here. A weighted sum of Zernike polynomials is said to be a "Zernike expansion," since it can be expanded into a list of its constituent basis functions. That is to say, each basis function, together with its "weight," is an addend to make up the sum. Moreover, when such a list or table is presented as a description of what went into making up a wavefront, we have a "Zernike spectrum," akin to a light spectrum that tells us how much of each wave length went into making up a given beam of light. In our context *the members of a Zernike spectrum are the constituent Zernike polynomials.*

✦

55. It appears that the H-S sensor is merely a very complicated spot retinoscope, capable of multiple simultaneous "mini-retinoscopies," depending on the number of lenslets (described later). An obvious question then is why bother with such a complicated method for refracting. The answer is that a standard refraction provides only a limited amount of information; it usually only addresses two aberrations, myopia/hyperopia and astigmatism. For a more comprehensive assessment, adequate for modern refractive surgery, we need to "refract" other additional modes. It turns out that most eyes have multiple aberrations, especially if they are diseased or have had surgery, which is why wavefronts are usually so complex and must be "decomposed" or "analyzed" into many constituent aberrations; recall paragraph 50. "Constituent" means "present" in this case.

56. The opposite is also feasible. Mathematically speaking, we can add together all the aberrations in an eye and arrive at the total refractive status; this procedure is called "synthesis." [6] That is to say, the overall refractive error is the synthesis of many simpler errors. Actually, summing and decomposing refractive errors are elementary, as we routinely add optical Rx's together (e.g., after over-refraction) and we can separate any sphero-cylindrical error into two independent Rx's.

57. Zernike polynomials are each mathematically independent; in technical terms they are mutually "orthogonal." We need not delve into the subtleties of orthogonality, but it does allow the independent addition of Zernike polynomials into a sum. (See Note 4 on page 89 for mathematical details.) Such independence also allows the analysis of an overall refractive error into its constituent Zernike polynomials, so that we can isolate each aberration and study it separately, including with regard to how much of each aberration the eye possesses.

58. This point serves to emphasize the distinction between (1) individual Zernike polynomials each of which represents one kind of aberration, and (2) the sum of Zernike polynomials which represents the overall refractive error and the total aberration of an ametropic eye. In other words we can speak of one particular component of the shape of a wavefront, which is independently described by a Zernike polynomial, and we can speak of the overall complete shape of a wavefront, which houses the weighted sum of many polynomials.

---

[6] The terms "synthesis" and "analysis" are more commonly used in Fourier's system, but are quite useful for Zernike's. We will cover details of the terminology later.

59. We now consider a very important question, recalling the issue raised in paragraph 47: If Zernike polynomials are predefined descriptions which only *identify* certain aberrations, and if they can be added together, where does the *magnitude* of each aberration enter into the picture? In other words, since eyes obviously vary with respect to the amount—read "diopters"—of each constituent refractive error, how does Zernike's system accommodate (pun intended) such variation?

60. The implication is that two questions and two tasks arise in order to make use of the Zernike polynomials. One is to decode *which* pre-defined Zernike polynomials pertain in a particular case. The other is to decode the *amount* of each Zernike polynomial that pertains, which means to calculate the magnitude of each aberration that is present in this case. The separation of these tasks is somewhat artificial in that both can be accomplished as one mathematical procedure, but the results appear as two separate parts in many equations and, more importantly, in clinical evaluations.

61. The cardinal pertinent principle, to which we already alluded, is that the sum of Zernike polynomials which represents the overall refractive error is a "*weighted sum.*" This is a mathematical way of stating that the sum allows each Zernike polynomial to have a "weight" which corresponds to the amount or magnitude of that aberration within the overall aberration. The "weight" is contained in a very important quantity called a "coefficient," and each Zernike polynomial is multiplied by that coefficient as it enters into the sum. We will see the equation for this weighted sum later. The coefficient is usually labeled by the letter "C" or less often by an "a." The units for coefficients are usually microns.

Suffice it now that each "coefficient-and-Zernike polynomial" term (called a "Zernike prescription") for the amount of, say, three diopters of myopia corresponds to "-3 D." In short, coefficients quantify Zernike polynomials and thus quantify aberrations (modes).

62. We are now in a position to see an algorithm for handling our data:

1. We gather data about a wavefront with a H-S device, which means we measure displacements of spots on a reference plane for this eye.

2. These displacements are converted to local slopes.

3. The overall shape of the wavefront is reconstructed from the assembly of slopes (in effect from the assembly of local altitudes). The word "overall" may be omitted in this context.

4. We decode which aberrations exist in this wavefront, which means we find which Zernike polynomials go into describing the wavefront of this eye.

5. We decode how much of each aberration goes into the wavefront. In effect, we find the "weight" of each aberration.

6. Steps 4 and 5 together, which form Zernike analysis, give us clinically relevant information about the optical status.

63. We note that steps 2 and 3 constitute the *reconstruction* of the wavefront aberration function, as completed in paragraph 43. Though there is overlap, the subsequent steps, 4 and 5, constitute the *analysis* of the wavefront aberration function into its constituent weighted Zernike polynomials. We will examine this complicated process shortly.

✦

64. At this juncture we turn to individual Zernike polynomials. As a working example, we select an aberration, *tilt*. The term "tilt" correctly implies that the wavefront is tilted ("tipped"). A counterpart of such tilting may be prismatic deviation, so it is not really a refractive error. However, tilt is a simple mode that lends itself to illustrating many details about Zernike polynomials.

Of course prisms induce other aberrations, notably chromatic, but these do not affect clinical optics in the context of refractive surgery. Though not common issues in routine refractive surgery, malpositioned intraocular lenses and corneal buttons may also involve tilt. For the moment, as we said, we are interested in tilt because it is sufficiently representative of Zernike polynomials in general.

65. We recall that aberrations displace the spots on the reference plane of a H-S device. Earlier we saw an example with just one spot. In the following case we will consider several spots, though for simplicity four will suffice, and we will ignore centroids and subapertures. Again the situation is best studied using a Cartesian system of coordinates. If the tilt happens to be in the x direction and the amount of displacement is Δx, then we would see all spots shifted in the x direction by the amount Δx. Assuming pure tilt in the x direction, there would be no Δy's. (If an aberration also involves a displacement in the y direction, we would see spots shifted by the amount Δy.) We can look inside a H-S sensor and see the shift of the four spots, and we can determine the amount of shift in units of distance such as millimeters or microns.

66. *These items of information—that the spots are shifted equally in the same direction and that they are shifted by a certain amount—is all we need to know; then we can identify the aberration as tilt, and we can quantify it.* We can also give it a more clinical name, e.g., "prism." And if we wished to remedy this aberration with refractive surgery, we have most of the essential information.

67. A diagram follows, comparing no aberration with a case of tilt.

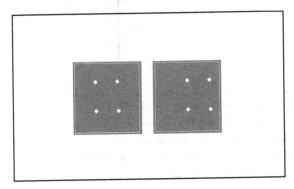

Views of a reference plane with four spots. For realism, the spots are bright and the reference plane is dark.

The left side is the appearance of the reference plane in absence of aberrations.

The right side is when the wavefront is tilted.

68. A term for the Δx-Δy data (paragraph 31) is the "variance." Later we will define this term more exactly, but for now we can use it to designate the overall displacements of the spots as they are detected by a H-S sensor. *If the wavefront reveals no aberrations, there will be no variance between the observed spots of light and the expected locations of those spots; all Δx's and all Δy's are zero.* In general a higher variance indicates a worse aberration, and higher variances are reflected in higher values for coefficients (as in paragraph 170 for a preview).

69. Because of the mathematics used to interpret the results, we say that—again with no aberrations—the *flat* wavefront has *no* slope. (Recall paragraph 12.) As we also mentioned (paragraph 24) this means that the distance between any "x and y" location on the wavefront and its corresponding "x and y" location on the reference plane should be the exactly same. In short, the wave front and reference plane should be parallel.

This cannot be the case in the presence of tilt. The *tilted* wavefront *does* have a slope; in fact it has the same slope "everywhere," as one edge of the wavefront is farther from the reference plane than the opposite edge. As we have seen, we can calculate the slope of the wavefront as well as the distance between the wavefront and reference plane at any location. Since all locations show the same tilt (equal slopes), we surmise that no other aberrations are in play.

70. A diagram follows:

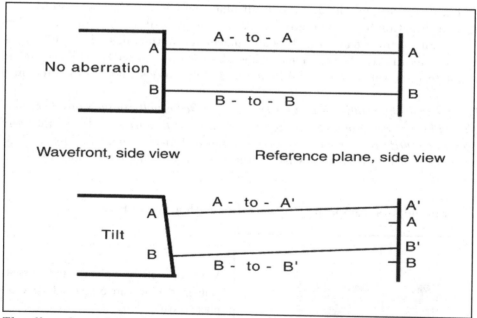

The effect of wavefront tilt on the location of spots on a reference plane. Tilt induces displacement of all spots (from A and B to A' and B') in one direction. The amount of displacement is the same for all spots. Without aberration, the wavefront is parallel to the reference plane; no wavefront error exists; A-to-A = B-to-B. With tilt, A-to-A' > B-to-B'. However, the tilt at A' equals tilt at B'.

71. At this juncture we have almost enough information to write out the Zernike polynomial for tilt in Cartesian coordinates. However, while these coordinates are convenient on the reference plane, it is better in general to use spherical polar coordinates. The reason is that these polynomials are better expressed in equations based on spherical polar coordinates. (We recall the unit circle in paragraph 22.) For this reason Zernike polynomials are said to be "circle polynomials." Because of their mathematical independence (paragraph 57) we also say that Zernike polynomials are "orthogonally defined inside a unit circle." This means that we should transform our x-y data into ρ-θ data, and that we should derive the Zernike polynomial in spherical polar coordinates.

72. Still, we should be aware that there are disadvantages to relying on spherical polar coordinates. Two problems deserve mention here. One is that spherical polar coordinates—along with the concept of a unit circle—presume that the pupil is truly round, which it rarely is. This means that when the pupil is not fully round, points that fall outside a perfect circle cannot be used in the calculations. The other problem is that with spherical coordinates centration is critical, which introduces a technical complication.

73. Let us now use an analogy to construct and write out the Zernike polynomial for tilt in spherical polar coordinates. Here we must be imaginative: We walk around the base of the Leaning Tower of Pisa, though we can call it a "tilted" tower. At every step we measure how high the first floor is from the ground.

We start at the northern side where this floor is 2 meters above the ground, and we proceed around the tower toward the east, where more of the wall is exposed because of the tilt. There we find that this floor is 2.5 meters off the ground, and then as we continue the floor becomes even higher. (The real Tower of Pisa does not tilt exactly one meter, but our analogy works better this way. [However it does tilt mainly west.])

We reach a point at the eastern side where the first floor is 3 meters off the ground, which is the maximum. Then as we turn toward the south, the height of the floor decreases back to 2 meters at the southern side, and still further it is only 1.5 meters off the ground until it reaches a minimum of 1 meter at the western side. Then we return to where we began. See the second diagram on page 27 and imagine it is the base of a tilted tower.

74. Now here is the interesting part. If we make a graph of our measurements as we complete the circle, *we will generate a sine curve, a.k.a a sine wave.* Obviously if the tilt had been worse, the amplitude of the sine wave—the extent of the up and down swings—would have been greater. Moreover if the tower were wider (if the radius of its floors were longer), our sine wave would also have a greater amplitude.

We further note that as we progressed around the building, we swept an angle of 360° (0° to 90° going from the northern side to the eastern side, etc.). As is often preferred, such a go-around can also be expressed in radians rather than degrees, in which case one cycle ("once around") is 2π radians. Thus progressing to 90° is equivalent to reaching $\pi/2$ radians, reaching 180° is equivalent to π radians, etc. We can label the radius of the tower as ρ. In any case, here is a graph of these results of our walk.

75. A diagram follows on the next page.

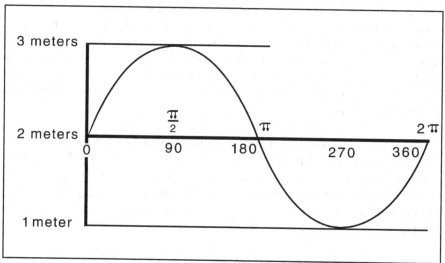

Sine curve generated while "walking around" a tilted tower. "Once around" is 360° or 2π radians. At 0 (zero), the floor is 2 meters off the ground. At 90 degrees the floor is 3 meters off the ground, etc. The amplitude is 2 meters.

76. Here is our conclusion: By applying basic trigonometry we have found that *if the radius of the building we circumscribed is* ρ *and the angle at any point in our walk-around is* θ, *then the tilted floor is described by the term "(ρ) (sin θ)."* In short, in spherical polar coordinates the polynomial

$$\rho \sin \theta$$

describes this tilt. Meanwhile, in this analogy tilt represents an aberration, and indeed "ρ sin θ " is the main component of the polar form of the Zernike polynomial for tilt. (In this exercise we concentrated on "sin θ." We will focus on "ρ" later. Also "ρ sin θ " is incomplete; it lacks a constant which we will soon provide, but it is not essential here.)

77. We should have a clear grasp of the very important concept that *a refractive error—an aberration—can be represented by a shape, specifically by a shape of the wavefront, and that this shape can be represented by a mathematical entity, specifically a Zernike polynomial.* (It can also be represented by a Fourier polynomial, as we will see later.) In this case "ρ *sin* θ " *is the mathematical description of the shape of the wavefront when the (sole) aberration is tilt.*

78. For the sake of argument, what is the mathematical description in *x*-coordinates of the shape of the wavefront which is cuboidal? The answer is x^3. And what is the mathematical description in ρθ-coordinates of the shape of the wavefront which is tilted? As we saw, the answer is ρ sin θ. At the risk of repetition, let us say this as a dialog:

"Describe a cubic shape." (Cartesian coordinates are easier for this purpose.)

"x^3."

"Write the Zernike polynomial if an aberration makes the wavefront is cuboidal."[7]

"x^3."

"Draw a picture of the shape described by the Zernike polynomial x^3."

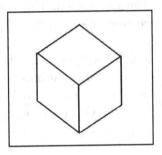

A cube, representing a possible shape for a wavefront.

"Now describe a *tilted shape*." (Polar coordinates are easier for this purpose.)

"$\rho \sin \theta$."

"Write the Zernike polynomial if an aberration (prism) made the wavefront tilted."

"$\rho \sin \theta$."

"Draw a picture of the shape described by the Zernike polynomial $\rho \sin \theta$."

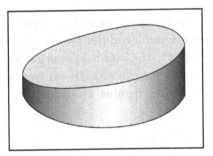

The shape of a wavefront in the presence of tilt.

This shape is described by the Zernike polynomial $\rho \sin \theta$.

We will return to this theme, particularly in regard to the role of shapes of wavefronts.

79. Though we have generated a sine curve, it helps to know that sine and cosine curves (also known as sine and cosine waves) are closely interrelated. They are both "sinusoidal." If we start our circumnavigation from a zero pont, the result is a sine wave; if we start further along, the result is a cosine wave. (Think of two walkers encircling the tilted tower: the "sine" walker starts at the west side; the "cosine" walker starts at the south side. Otherwise, the routes are similar.) Therefore, the difference between sines and cosines is a matter of phase. By custom, a graphed sine wave starts at $x = 0$ and $y = 0$, whereas the analogous cosine wave starts a quarter wavelength further along the x axis; they are "out of step" or out of phase by one quarter of the complete cycle, but both are sinusoidal.

---

[7] Of course this is in theory only. No natural wavefront is ever cuboidal.

80.   To make full use of this exercise we must agree on which way to "walk around" the wavefront (clockwise or counterclockwise), on where the prime meridian for angle θ is located (zero θ is generally the positive y coordinate), and on when a value is positive or negative. We will see that whether the Zernike polynomial contains a sine or cosine is determined by the direction of the tilt; i.e., in the y-direction or the x-direction. This convention is quite logical; the polynomial has a sine part if the tilt is such that $x = 0$ and $y = 0$, etc.

In any case the curve is "sinusoidal," and it is called a "sinusoid." As we said, the range for θ is zero to 360 degrees, though it is commonly expressed in radians, so that in most equations θ is between zero and 2π. The angle θ is the "meridional angle." (We also recall from the definition of a unit circle that ρ ranges from zero to 1. This provision simplifies the comparison of various wavefronts.)

81.   In the "walk-around" we observed one complete sine wave, encountering one maximum and one minimum. This is not always the case; some aberrations are such that we observe *more than one complete sinusoidal wave* in one "walk-around." The number of waves we observe appears in the Zernike polynomials as a number in front of the angle θ. This number is called the "meridional frequency" or the "sinusoidal frequency" or the "azimuthal frequency." We prefer "meridional." (Navigators will associate azimuthal angles with compass bearings.)

82.   For instance even simple astigmatism is complex enough so that it has a meridional frequency of at least 2; imagine walking once around a saddle; two maxima and two minima. In the usual way the system is set up, the "index" (the number) is negative when it describes meridional frequency in its sine phase. The index for the meridional frequency is not written if it is 1. Here is such a polynomial, representing regular astigmatism, with a meridional frequency of two:

$$\rho^2 \cos 2\theta.$$

Again let us be clear: "$\rho^2 \cos 2\theta$" is the mathematical description of the shape of the wavefront when the eye is beset by simple astigmatism. (If we wish to "grind" an astigmatic wavefront the way we would manufacture a cylindrical trial lens using modern automated machinery, "$\rho^2 \cos 2\theta$" will appear in the equation we would enter.)

A glance ahead at the table of polynomials in paragraph 93 will show other examples, including ones with no sin or cos terms. These are quite simple; they "look the same (no rise or fall of the level of the floor) as we walk around them."

83.   We can use the description of astigmatism to conclude the theme introduced in paragraph 77, namely the addition or summation of shapes. In paragraph 78 we saw what the wavefront might look like from an eye with tilt (though tilt is not a typical refractive error), and on page 29 is a diagram of a wavefront from an eye with simple astigmatism. This shape is usually said to resemble a saddle, or a warped surface with two high points and two low points.

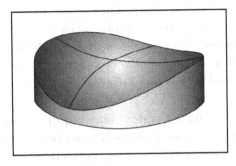

The shape of a wavefront in the presence of (simple) astigmatism.

This shape is described by the Zernike polynomial $\rho^2 \cos 2\theta$.

Now let us amalgamate the two aberrations, tilt and astigmatism, by considering the wavefront from an eye with both. In other words let us add the two shapes together.

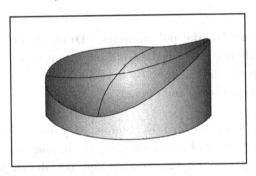

Shape of a wavefront in the presence of *tilt and astigmatism*.

The surface is tilted *and* warped.

We emphasize that this wavefront shows both structural features. It has the shape of tilt plus the shape of astigmatism, and here we apply the principle cited in paragraph 57 that Zernike polynomials are independent and can be added to each other. We will see the algebra later and, more practically, we will be able to work backwards. We will start with an overall wavefront as above and decode its constituent shapes—which means that we can analyze which aberrations are present in an eye.

We also skimmed over the issue of quantity—how much tilt and how much astigmatism—as we did in paragraph 61, where we only mentioned coefficients; we will return to this issue.

84.   We note again that wavefronts—shaped by the overall refractive errors—are sums of constituent shapes. Zernike polynomials—associated with individual refractive errors—describe these constituent shapes. We can add polynomials to reconstruct entire complex wavefronts. To emphasize this key point, as it is so important in practice, we reiterate that we can start with complex wavefronts as determined by H-S devices and then analyze them into simpler but weighted polynomial ingredients.

85.   The above example can serve to look ahead at a key difference between the Zernike system and the Fourier system. In the former, words like "astigmatism" conjure up definite and familiar clinical entities. The mathematical descriptions of the constituents may be complicated—the Zernike polynomials may be intricate mathematical terms—but what they stand for is clearly documented.

The Fourier approach foregoes clinically familiar constituents in favor of basic geometric shapes which are built out of simple waves (called wavelets). On the one hand, this system makes the corresponding Fourier polynomial comparatively simple. (The Fourier system also entails polynomials, even in this context.) On the other hand few of us can look at a Fourier polynomial and automatically associate it with a particular refractive error. In fact a separate system is needed to link Fourier polynomials with words like astigmatism, myopia, etc.

Moreover, the mathematical descriptions in the Fourier system may require a larger number of smaller polynomials. By analogy, Fourier would not just analyze wavefronts in terms of shapes; he would "decompose" them into their (curved) lines. The trade-off then is as follows: The Fourier system analyzes wavefronts into numerous simpler geometric constituents which can readily accommodate any possible case, but these constituents have no clinically familiar counterparts.

86. Let us go back to the basics about Zernike polynomials. Once we know how the polynomial for tilt is constructed, other aberrations can be similarly approached. Of course Zernike polynomials describe more complex aberrations, such as various forms of defocus, various forms of astigmatism, spherical aberrations, and comas.

Moreover, certain likely combinations are represented by blends of polynomials, such as defocus and astigmatism, tilt and coma, defocus and spherical aberration, and others; later we will see why. Other modes, mostly unrecognized until this technology was developed, are not identified by name but are nevertheless represented by polynomials.

◆

87. This is an opportune juncture for a brief review. We can think of Zernike polynomials as follows. We have at our disposal an inventory of shapes which represent various optical aberrations. The mathematical descriptions of these shapes are polynomials, and they can be added together in various combinations to represent the more complex shapes of human wavefronts. These complex shapes describe overall refractive errors. That is to say, an optical state is represented by a complex shape. Conversely, we can analyze a complex shape to determine which constituent shapes are included. Once we say it, the concept is surprisingly simple: Zernike analysis is finding appropriate shapes within a compendium of shapes. The detected shapes correspond to the eye's constituent refractive errors.

Let us be clear about the basic idea behind Zernike (and, as we shall see, Fourier) analysis: *Analysis answers the question, "what is in a wavefront."* By that we mean which polynomials describe the shape of the wavefront. The idea is not all exotic or esoteric. Assume you have 95 cents. We might ask, "what coins are in your pocket?" You reach in and find two dimes and three quarters. You have performed analysis! We will use this analogy later.

◆

88. This approach has a drawback, one which is both practically significant and instructive. We will find that a Zernike system is "prepared" for a wavefront that has two structural features, a bump (convexity) on the left and a dip (concavity) on the right. In other words, the system's inventory of shapes includes one constituent with a bump and dip. However, to deal with a case with *only one of these features*, such as just the bump, the system nevertheless first calls upon the polynomial which includes both features. Then the system applies a polynomial for a "negative dip" on the right, so as to cancel—to subtract out—the non-existent dip.

Unfortunately, this second polynomial might describe a shape with a third feature (e.g., a warp) which is not present in this case. Therefore the system needs to use yet another polynomial for the third shape to cancel out this nonexistent feature, etc. Think of describing just a mountain if you only have the descriptive phrase "mountain and valley." You are forced to say, "mountain with valley, but minus the valley." Obviously, the entire procedure may be very cumbersome, but the consolation is that the inventory of shapes can handle just about any possibility, and the necessary mathematics functions well despite the ostensibly illogical approach.

89. In a clinical setting, the issue in the previous paragraph arises with respect to the Zernike polynomial for coma, particularly in the measurement of an eye which has an ectasia or keratoconus. Coma in effect consists of a bulge in one half of the wavefront and a dip in the other half, whereas keratoconus or ectasias need *not* be accompanied by a dip in the wavefront. The Zernike algorithm will detect such an aberration but will report it as a coma. Then, since there is no concavity, the algorithm will invoke the mode for another aberration, one which the eye does not really have, in order to cancel out the concavity.

90. A similar chain of events might follow in dealing with a localized flat corneal scar. This defect might be interpreted by a Zernike algorithm as a coma-*sans*-bulge, which entails a cancellation of the bulge by another mode, etc. (How did these complications develop historically? Because in effect Zernike's system was devised for telescopes and microscopes which do not suffer from isolated ectasias or scars, so that modes for these were not included. See footnote on page 65.)

91. We note how one Zernike polynomial can cancel parts of another polynomial. This means that polynomials are not only added to each other; they can be mathematically subtracted from each other; one mode can undo parts of another mode. Indeed we will encounter equations with negative terms, signifying that shapes can be negative and that negative shapes at some location can cancel positive ones in the same location.

On the other hand the same issues and complications apply in Fourier systems, but there the processes are less cumbersome since each polynomial is simpler and all are basically the same. We will revisit this point, as it represents a technical advantage of Fourier systems.

The LISTING and STRUCTURE of ZERNIKE POLYNOMIALS

92. We are ready for a list—a compendium or inventory—of Zernike polynomials. This particular list is organized by means of a single-index system in which the polynomials are numbered consecutively. These indices are usually called "mode numbers"; these appear in the first column. However, the sequence is not universally agreed upon; this one is arranged in the approximate order of complexity, but other means of enumeration exist.

Here the list includes 24 polynomials, though it could be much longer, since it is possible to identify and measure more than 60 different aberrations. (In theory the list could be infinitely long.) However, our list excludes the normalization constants, since these are not essential at the moment. It is also wise to keep in mind that each member of this list is the mathematical description of a shape, while the wavefront of a particular eye is built out of a weighted sum of a group of these shapes.

93. The single-index list of Zernike polynomials appears below and continues on the next page:

Mode Number	Zernike Polynomial in Polar (Radial) Form	Name of Polynomial; clinical name of mode
1	$\rho \cos \theta$	Tilt in x-direction
2	$\rho \sin \theta$	Tilt in y-direction
3	$2\rho^2 - 1$	Defocus (Power)
4	$\rho^2 \cos 2\theta$	Defocus + astigmatism 45/135
5	$\rho^2 \sin 2\theta$	Defocus + astigmatism 90/180
6	$(3\rho^2 - 2)\rho \cos \theta$	Tilt + horiz. coma along x axis
7	$(3\rho^2 - 2)\rho \sin \theta$	Tilt + vertical coma along y axis
8	$6\rho^4 - 6\rho^2 + 1$	Defocus + spherical aberration
9	$\rho^3 \cos 3\theta$	Trefoil in x-direction
10	$\rho^3 \sin 3\theta$	Trefoil in y-direction
11	$(4\rho^2 - 3)\rho^2 \cos 2\theta$	More complex aberrations are
12	$(4\rho^2 - 3)\rho^2 \sin 2\theta$	usually not named.
13	$(10\rho^4 - \rho^2 + 3)\rho \cos \theta$	
14	$(10\rho^4 - \rho^2 + 3)\rho \sin \theta$	
15	$20\rho^6 - 30\rho^4 + 12\rho^2 - 1$	

16	$\rho^4 \cos 4\theta$	
17	$\rho^4 \sin 4\theta$	
18	$(5\rho^2 - 4)\rho^3 \cos 3\theta$	
19	$(5\rho^2 - 4)\rho^3 \sin 3\theta$	
20	$(15\rho^4 - 20\rho^2 + 6)\rho^2 \cos 2\theta$	
21	$(15\rho^4 - 20\rho^2 + 6)\rho^2 \sin 2\theta$	
22	$(35\rho^6 - 60\rho^4 + 30\rho^2 - 4)\rho \cos\theta$	
23	$(35\rho^6 - 60\rho^4 + 30\rho^2 - 4)\rho \sin\theta$	
24	$70\rho^8 - 140\rho^6 + 90\rho^4 - 20\rho^2 + 1$	

94. Most of the Zernike polynomials in this list are expressed using a spherical polar system of coordinates, which is the most mathematically elegant way. However, as is sometimes more intuitive, the directions of prism and coma are given in Cartesian terms, whereby x is horizontal and y is vertical. As a comparison, in the case of defocus and astigmatism, $\rho^2 \cos 2\theta$ in spherical polar form would be the same as $(x^2 - y^2)$ in Cartesian form.

95. With this list at hand, we now turn to a detailed study of the mathematical structure of typical Zernike polynomials, including elements we skimmed over so far. While this and subsequent topics are of necessity mainly mathematical, they reveal important principles and commonly encountered terminology. (Admittedly, mathematicians and optical engineers may object to some of my shortcuts.)

96. Each Zernike polynomial consists of three parts, customarily presented in the following manner:

    1.   A constant, the "normalization constant."

    2.   A "radial-dependent polynomial" or "radial function."

    3.   A "sine-cosine term" or "sinusoidal function."

97. As a preview, here is an example showing the three parts explicitly. This is polynomial 18 in the above list, but now the normalization constant is included:

$\sqrt{12}$	$(5\rho^2 - 4)\rho^3$	$\cos 3\theta$

Though it breaks the algebraic sequence, it is easier to save the discussion of normalization constants for last. We now take up the radial function.

98.   The "radial" function in the second box depends only on the radius, expressed as ρ, which is one of the two dimensions in polar coordinates. (We recall that ρ is the radial distance normalized in a unit circle so as to vary between zero and 1, no matter what the size of the pupil and wavefront.) The radial function reveals how the shape of the wavefront changes along the radius; imagine how the altitude which changes walking along a radius of a round mountain from the center out, except the maximum radius is 1. More on this analogy shortly.

99.   The radial function is the only true polynomial part of a Zernike polynomial. It has a ρ more than once, each ρ may be raised to a power (an exponent), and each may be preceded by a number (5 in the above case). For clarity we will call each such number (e.g., 5) a "factor," because it is important but it is not part of the normalization constant. For positive identification, the radial function (with its factors) can be labeled by R with a superscript and subscript, e.g., R_n^m . We will explain the n and m later, but the radial function can be calculated from the values of n and m.

100.   At this point we must detour for an important definition: the term "order." This term is borrowed from algebra, where it has several meanings. In our context "order" has an exact mathematical definition which we will see in paragraph 117, but in general *order is a very useful expression of the complexity of a Zernike polynomial.*

Indeed Zernike polynomials—and the aberrations they describe—can be organized into a hierarchy based on orders, reminiscent of the periodic table of elements. However, this hierarchy forms a pyramid-shaped table. Each line of this table contains polynomials and corresponding aberrations (modes) of one *order*, and the members of each order are closely related. The orders are numbered from zero up, though the lowest ("zero-eth") order has no clinical significance. For a preview, an example of such a pyramid-shaped table of Zernike polynomials appears in paragraph 130. It is an alternative to the single-index list.

The first significant order is tilt, the simplest aberration. Members of the second order—the "second-order" Zernike polynomials—are particularly important, in that they are equivalent to the familiar sphero-cylindrical aberrations measured in ordinary refraction. Aberrations beyond this level—"third-order" aberrations and higher ones, which are even more complex—are all "high-order" aberrations (HOA's), each of which is described by a high-order polynomial. In effect, any Rx which is not addressed simply by sphere, cylinder and axis is "high-order." Conversely, "low order" aberrations are of the first and second order, even though tilt is rarely a concern in refractive surgery.

The importance of high-order aberrations is clear: We can measure them with modern equipment (e.g., aberrometers); they occur naturally (e.g., irregular astigmatism), pathologically (e.g., keratoconus) and iatrogenically (e.g., after corneal surgery); and we have the tools to treat them.

The highest power—the largest exponent of ρ—in the radial function matches the order, though this is not always apparent because of the way functions may be written. (For example mode 11 in paragraph 93 $[(4\rho^2 - 3)\rho^2 \cos 2\theta]$ is 4th-order, since ρ's exponents [2, 2] are added together in multiplication.) The common symbol for order is "n" as in the label R_n^m (paragraph 99).

35

35

101. Let us focus on the factors associated with each ρ of the radial function, though in many cases these factors are 1 (one) and therefore are not written out. We can look at the principles surrounding these factors first in an empiric way in the following example, a high-order Zernike polynomial.

$$70\,\rho^8 - 140\,\rho^6 + 90\,\rho^4 - 20\,\rho^2 + 1.$$

This example is selected for its comparative simplicity, and it appears as item 24 in the table in paragraph 93. We still omit the normalization constant here so as not to complicate the presentation.

102. Next, we focus on just the factors, omitting the ρ's but retaining their + and −signs. We note that when we add these factors together, they add up to 1. Thus,

$$70 - 140 + 90 - 20 + 1 = 1.$$

103. Let us on purpose ignore the last value, + 1. We can do so since the Zernike polynomial for the "piston" is 1, but this aberration is clinically meaningless.[8] In that case *the remaining factors add up to zero*:

$$70 - 140 + 90 - 20 = 0.$$

104. Now let us take a more analytic—though abbreviated—approach. The fact that the factors add up to zero (when we ignore the + 1) reflects the following concept: *Each Zernike polynomial, except for the zero-order "piston," must have a zero average (or zero mean).* We explain this idea next.

105. The wavefront is a disk-like surface in front of an eye. Any aberrations (except the "piston") may force parts of the wavefront to protrude anterior to this surface, and these aberrations may also force other parts of the wavefront to protrude posterior to this surface. In fact we can calculate these protrusions, forward and backward, in microns; they are wavefront errors. An example is coma, part of which appears as a forward bulge in the wavefront and part of which is a backward depression or concavity. Think of a circular island with a mountain and a canyon.

106. The point is this: The *average* of the protrusions, anterior and posterior, described by each Zernike polynomial (except piston) should lie on the same surface; the deformities ought to be centered in an agreed-upon frame of reference. In more technical words, the mean (average) of each Zernike polynomial (each mode except the zero mode) over the interior of the unit circle must be zero.

---

[8] The "piston" aberration arises in Zernike polynomials applied to astronomical telescopes. A shift of an optical component forward or backward (like a piston in a cylinder) is a serious defect in a telescope. The closest ophthalmic counterpart might be proptosis or enophthalmos, which also does not ordinarily call for refractive surgery.

This is a form of normalization, in the sense that the constants, such as 70, −140, + 90, and −20, together "normalize" the values of the Zernike polynomials to a zero mean (or zero average). Normalization is a mathematical device that adjusts data to allow them to make sense. A good example is in calculations of the probabilities of several events; when we ensure that all the probabilities add up to 100%, the constituent probabilities are said to be normalized. We already saw normalization applied so that all wavefronts have the same maximum radius, namely 1.

Though the notion of zero average for each polynomial is currently accepted, we could consider the wavefront error to be zero (not zero average, just zero) at the plane of the pupil. The latter convention, though rarely used, complicates the literature on items such as making models of wavefronts. Think again of a wavefront like an island with mountains and canyons; the more accepted convention implies that the *average* altitude is zero. The zero-at-pupil convention is akin to the idea of sea level, which is then considered to be where the *lowest* altitude is zero.

107.   We now consider the "sinusoidal" function (in the third box in paragraph 97) which depends on the angle θ. This angle is the other dimension in spherical polar coordinates. It is associated with—and is a function of—the meridional frequency *m*. Therefore, it is labeled as either $\rho \cos m\theta$ or $\rho \sin m\theta$. (See paragraph 81.) Since the sinusoidal feature of this term can be a sine or cosine, it can also be called the "sinusoidal/co-sinusoidal" term, though we rarely bother. A better alternative name is the "angular" part of a Zernike polynomial.

Incidentally, a reason for using spherical polar coordinates in this setting is so that the radial and sinusoidal function can be easily multiplied together to form Zernike polynomials (though this wording is not entirely accurate, since only the radial function is a true polynomial). Another fine point is that the applicability of the sinusoidal function requires that Zernike polynomials have "rotational symmetry," so that this function repeats itself after every complete rotation.

108.   We see that the sinusoidal function tells us how the shape of the wavefront changes *while sweeping out an angle*. We recall that the radial function tells us how the shape of the wavefront changes *along the radius*. Now we can reconsider the titled tower analogy: As we walked around its circumference, we swept out angle θ, and thus we experienced the sinusoidal function. We recorded our observations in a graph as in paragraph 75.

If instead we had walked along the floor of the tower from its center to its wall, we would have progressed along the radial distance ρ and we would have experienced the radial function. If we had recorded our observations in a diagram, we would have created a cross-section. These concepts will reappear when we compare the complexity of aberrations in detail. The message in this section is that we need both elements, "ρ" as well as "$\sin m\theta$," to describe tilt (as an example), though for simplicity we glossed over the former in the tower analogy. We mentioned *m* earlier because it appears in the label R_n^m; more on this later.

109.   Let us finally turn to the *normalization constants*. In the pattern above, the $\sqrt{12}$ in the first box is such a constant. Actually these constants are not essential for the integrity of the Zernike polynomials, but they are very helpful for the role the Zernike polynomials play in this setting. The purpose of normalizing constants is to force *all constituent Zernike polynomials together to have unit variance*. In other words it is beneficial to have the variance of each contributor to a wavefront be 1 when its coefficient is 1, because then all polynomials exert a balanced influence when added to each other or compared against each other. Hence we also say that every polynomial is "scaled" or "sized" by multiplication with a constant, so that all polynomials together in one eye have unit variance. (Each polynomial is also given a "weight" by its coefficient, but this is another ingredient to which we will return. Then we can define variance and unit variance more accurately.)

110. The two adjustments we just described, namely assuring "zero mean" and "unit variance," can be considered together, since both cooperate to place all modes in a common frame of reference and to allow effective comparisons between modes. In short, *Zernike polynomials (except piston) are scaled so that they have a zero mean and have unit variance.*

Incidentally, in Cartesian x-y-z coordinates, we can say that the unit-circle and zero-mean restrictions apply in the x and y dimensions while the unit variance restriction applies in the z dimension. Thus, no matter how severe the aberrations, the arena for Zernike polynomials is limited in all three dimensions. Though here the analogy is strained, think again of a wavefront as many mountains and canyons; we prefer that all the highs and lows balance each other so that they add up to 1 and that they fit into a circle of size 1.

111. The normalization constant is easy to calculate. Its equation has two variables, n, which is the "order" of Zernike polynomial, and m, which is the meridional frequency (as discussed in the next paragraph). Here is the equation for the normalization constant N:

$$N = \sqrt{\frac{2(n+1)}{1+\delta}} \ .$$

To be precise, it is only the radial function that needs normalization. On the other hand without normalization, the coefficient could not correctly show the amount of each aberration in a wavefront, so we often say that the normalization constant normalizes the entire mode.

112. The δ in the above equation represents a bit of mathematical minutia called the Kronecker delta function. Its value is 1 if m is zero (no meridional frequency and no sine/cosine are involved), and otherwise it is zero. The standard symbol for the normalization constant includes a superscript and subscript for positive identification, as in N_n^m. We note that a specific normalization constant is fixed to each Zernike polynomial; it does not vary. We also note that Zernike polynomials of higher order (larger n) and higher meridional frequency (larger m) receive a somewhat larger normalization constant. This is how the relative sizes of Zernike polynomials are evened out.

113. Omitting extraneous explanations, here are two Zernike polynomials from the list but with their associated normalization constants included:

$$\sqrt{6}\ \rho^2 \cos 2\theta \quad \text{and} \quad \sqrt{5}\ (6\rho^4 - 6\rho^2 + 1)\ .$$

114. Three more comments about these normalization constants are needed. First, again the terminology is beset by confusing alternatives. Sometimes normalization constants are called normalization "coefficients," but this word is better reserved for another important quantity. Normalization "factor" is also seen, but we use the term otherwise, as in paragraph 99.

115. Second, the number that appears before a θ is not part of the normalization constant, and it is not one of our "factors." It is the meridional frequency. The other numbers before the ρ's, which are our "factors," are not true normalization constants.

116. Third, more than one instance of normalization is in play. The creation of a unit circle in paragraph 22 is a kind of normalization, and the above-described normalization constant is another. Even causing a Zernike polynomial to average out to zero in a unit circle is a form of normalization.

◆

117. Let us now return to listing Zernike polynomials in another way than by a single index (as in paragraph 92). As said, Zernike polynomials can be characterized by two parameters, *order* and *meridional frequency*, which reside in two of their three mathematical parts (paragraph 96). This two-parameter system of identification allows the "double index" or "dual index" method of listing polynomials and parts of polynomials. A general example is the label for the radial function R_n^m, and we will say still more about the *n* and *m* shortly. The double index listing method is more informative than single index systems, mainly because the two indices reveal more about the *complexity of the particular aberration.*

118. Let us recall that the radial function in the polynomial tells us how the shape of the wavefront changes along the radius, and the sinusoidal function tells us how that shape changes along the circumference. These two processes correspond respectively to order and meridional frequency. We should keep in mind that both functions, the radial and the sinusoidal, are needed to describe the shape of a wavefront (basically because we describe the wavefront in two dimensions). We also need both parameters to better compare polynomials in terms of complexity.

119. We can still think of each polynomial's complexity in terms of terrain which has a number of peaks and valleys or mountains and canyons. The *order* is determined by the number of peaks and valleys we would encounter "walking" along a radius. These peaks and valleys are easy to depict on a cross-section of a model (as mentioned in paragraphs 98 and 108). Since such a cross-section is made by "cutting" the model along a diameter, each order is really a "radial order." In short, an order is the level of radial complexity. When order is specified by an index, its usual label is the subscript "*n*," which can only be positive. In general, each higher order (each *n* increased by 1) indicates one additional peak and valley on a radial cross-section.

120. The other parameter of complexity, the *meridional frequency*, is the number of peaks and valleys we would encounter going around the model (along its circumference rather than its radius; paragraphs 108 and 118). This numeral indicates circumferential complexity. For instance, regular astigmatism has a meridional of 2; imagine walking once around a saddle (rather than a tilted tower); we would encounter two "peaks" and two "valleys," which represent two maxima and two minima in a sine or cosine curve. See also paragraph 83, where we saw an astigmatic "warped" or "saddle-like" surface.

When the meridional frequency is specified by an index, its usual label is the superscript "*m*," though it can be positive or negative. (Depending on which custom is heeded, the *m* may be negative if it describes meridional frequency in its sine phase. The *m* can also be even or odd, making meridional frequency even more difficult to envision.) Here is a polynomial representing regular astigmatism, with a meridional frequency of two: $\rho^2 \cos 2\theta$. Its meridional index, 2, should be positive since it describes frequency in its cosine phase.

121. One use of the meridional frequency index *m* is to show how many modes (how many Zernike polynomials) share the same order (the same *n* index). Borrowing from biological taxonomy, meridional frequency identifies the "family" within an "order." In the above case, $\rho^2 \cos 2\theta$, regular astigmatism—which is a second-order aberration as shown by the exponent of ρ—can exist in two modes. The other mode is $\rho^2 \sin 2\theta$. Their *m* indices usually are (+)2 and −2 respectively.

122. In comparing order and meridional frequency, increased order of wavefronts means they are more uneven or irregular, particularly centrally, and increased frequency means that their edges are more "ruffled" or more "frilly." If the order is zero, there is no clinical aberration (only perhaps "piston"); the wavefront is flat. If order is one (1) there is tilt. If the meridional frequency of a significant aberration is zero, the aberration is spherically symmetrical (e.g., pure defocus or pure spherical aberration; refractive errors that have no axes) and it "looks the same—no ruffles—as we walk around it." As mentioned and as we will elaborate, a non-zero meridional frequency indicates that the aberration has some kind of angular direction, notably an axis. (Of course astigmatism is the prime instance.)

123. An important point is that one kind of aberration can have various levels of complexity and can reside in several orders. For example "regular" astigmatism is a second-order aberration, one that has its own Zernike polynomials. However, an eye can have a more complex higher-order astigmatism, which has its own more intricate polynomials. In our list includes several "astigmatisms," each of a higher order. (Three-axis astigmatism is a.k.a. "trefoil," etc. The meridional frequency of trefoil is 3.)

124. As the above discussion suggests, we can accurately delineate any polynomial just by means of its *n* and *m*. However, this may be easier with a model, diagram, or any suitable picture; e.g., in paragraph 83. Furthermore, we would have to memorize the meaning of each *n* and *m*; for example an *m* of some value would mean something different depending on whether it is even or odd. Finally, a verbal description of a very complicated (high-order) polynomial would be of little practical value. A better use of these indices is to fashion a double-index list and to associate each pair of indices (for a relatively simple instance) with a picture of the shape described by the corresponding polynomial.

40

125.   Not only does the system of classifying Zernike polynomials by order and meridional frequency allow each aberration to have a unique mathematical designation, but this system also allows unambiguous associations between the parts of a Zernike polynomial. For instance the normalization constant N_2^3 goes only with the radial polynomial R_2^3, and both belong to the Zernike polynomial Z_2^3. In this case, the meridional frequency, m, is 3; the order, n, is 2.

126.   The information from the foregoing several paragraphs can be expressed and summarized in two equations which differ for cosine vs. sine functions. These key equations (spread out to show the terms) appear in one form of another in most detailed sources on Zernike polynomials:

$$Z_n^m(\rho, \theta) = N_n^m R_n^{|m|}(\rho) \cos m\theta \quad if \ m \geq 0,$$

$$Z_n^m(\rho, \theta) = -N_n^m R_n^{|m|}(\rho) \sin m\theta \quad if \ m < 0.$$

These equations are not as formidable as they appear. In words, Zernike polynomials are identified by two indices, n and m. Each Zernike polynomial is the product of three values: a normalization constant N which is identified by the same two indices; a radial function R identified by these two indices (except the +/− sign of m does not matter; hence $|m|$); and a sinusoidal function, if any. The sinusoidal function can be a cosine or sine and it depends on the radius ρ and on m. The radial function gives the shape of the wavefront along its radius. The sinusoidal function gives the shape along the circumference. The normalization constant centers the shape.

127.   So much for the preliminaries. We can now look at an example of the double index format for listing some Zernike polynomials. This format of course includes the two indices for identifying the polynomials, and it may also show their respective coefficients and other parts (normalization constants and radial terms). Each row holds one order, marked by the subscript n. In each row the superscript gives the meridional frequency, given by the superscript m. Again, positive m's (+m) indicate a cosine function and negative m's (−m) indicate a sine function.

128.   Despite efforts to ensure uniformity, alternative conventions create some confusion. However, in general Zernike polynomials are identified through the following double index (or two index or dual index) template, on which most experts agree:

$$Z_n^{\pm m}$$

For any given n (which means within any order) m can only be equal to −n, or −n +2, or −n +4, or −n +6, etc. Since n can be, say, 2, some m's can be zero, as occurs when the polynomial is spherically symmetric. However n and m are only whole numbers, never fractions.

The custom about the correlation between cosine/sine and positive/negative superscripts is tied to how pairs of polynomials such as Z_2^{-2} and Z_2^2 indicate axes; we will return to this important arrangement later.

129. Most double-index formats present the polynomials in a pyramid, the apex of which is given to a single mode, the zero-order "piston," even though it is clinically unimportant. Below the apical zero-eth order, the first row holds the two first-order Zernike polynomials for tilt. The second row holds the three second-order Zernike polynomials for defocus and regular astigmatism. The members in this row describe the familiar sphero-cylindrical Rx, the only aberrations generally accessible to ordinary refraction (and amenable to spectacle or contact lens "correction"). We note the subscript 2 in every polynomial in this row. The third row holds the four third-order Zernike polynomials, etc.

The "Zernike pyramid" shown below stops at the fourth order, and because the base widens progressively, most readable renditions stop at six. (Zernike analysis beyond six orders may be superfluous anyway, because it does not significantly affect the clinical outcomes in most cases.)

130. The usual "Zernike pyramid" then looks like this:

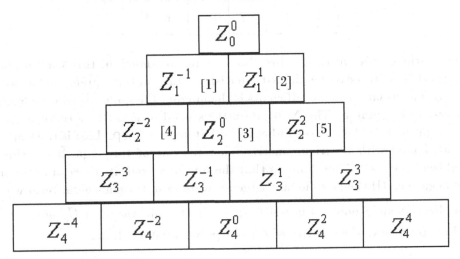

The superscripts and subscripts identify each polynomial, and several single-index numbers are shown in the bracket. The latter refer to the mode numbers in the list in paragraph 93, but the correlation becomes complicated for higher orders because various conventions exit. I.e., a logical and orderly listing in a column may be non-consecutive in a pyramid, as is apparent in the second row. (This occurs because, for instance, defocus is represented by a polynomial which is less complex than the two kinds of astigmatism and is therefore often listed before astigmatism in a columnar presentation. However, in a pyramidal format the logical sequence in one row is astigmatism-defocus-other astigmatism. Thus, the simpler polynomial is winged by two more complex ones on either side.) As mentioned, a more useful point is this: In the typical Zernike pyramid, the third row—which constitutes the second order—houses basic myopia-hyperopia-astigmatism. *All subsequent rows hold high-order aberrations.*

Incidentally, equations allow the calculation of the single index from the order and the meridional indices. Oftentimes "*j*" (or "*i*") is used for the single index, in which case we see

$$j = \frac{n(n+2)+m}{2}$$, and similar but reverse equations allow *n* and *m* to be extracted from *j*.

131. We emphasize that each cell in the pyramid holds a unique Zernike polynomial whose main parameters of complexity are discernable from the information held by the two indices, and this scheme applies to several parts of the polynomial. Thus for the polynomial labeled " Z_2^{-2} " in the pyramid, a complete expression which includes its coefficient is

$$\text{``}\ C_2^{-2}\ N_2^{-2}\ R_2^{-2}\,(\rho)\ \sin 2\,\theta.\ \text{''}$$

The same superscripts and subscripts connect the coefficient C_2^{-2} to the other parts unambiguously. Clearly, this expression is of the second order (subscript) with meridional frequency -2 (superscript).

132. Therefore, the entire pattern for a complete Zernike polynomial (a Zernike prescription) could be, for example,

0.6	$\sqrt{6}$	$\rho^{\,2}$	$\sin 2\,\theta$

The C term—the coefficient (in the first box)—tells how much of this kind of aberration is present in this eye, in this case regular astigmatism. (Many authors prefer an "a" as a label for coefficients.) The usual unit for coefficients is the micron, though units of wavelength of light and diopters are acceptable. The N term (in the second box) is the normalization constant. The R term (in the third box) is the radial term that depends on ρ. Last is the sinusoidal term (in the fourth box) with its trigonometric function, sine of the angle θ in this case; the meridional frequency is 2. This 2 means that the sine curve repeats twice, and the superscript should be negative. (If the meridional frequency were zero, the sinusoidal term would simply be 1 by implication and would not be written). In short, while the term C_2^{-2} gives its quantity, the last three terms give the identity of Zernike polynomial itself; i.e.,

$$Z_2^{-2}\ =\ N_2^{-2}\ R_2^{-2}\,(\rho)\ \sin 2\,\theta.$$

133. However, despite the common use of this scheme, there is no universal agreement on precisely what constitutes a Zernike polynomial. Mathematicians may point out that only the radial function or radial term is really a polynomial. Less meticulous experts say that the radial and meridional terms together form a Zernike polynomial but without the normalization constant, since it is not essential. Others include the normalization constant because it is needed for unit variance. Finally, some authors include the coefficient as well, since it quantifies the aberration; i.e., a Zernike polynomial then is a coefficient multiplied by a normalization constant, a radial function, and a sinusoidal function.

We need not bother with these nuances; suffice it that all mathematical terms of Zernike polynomials participate in describing optical aberrations. That is to say, all parts of a particular Zernike polynomial characterize a particular shape which may be a feature of a wavefront.

WEIGHTED SUMS and a FUNDAMENTAL ZERNIKE EQUATION

134.   Earlier we equated the coefficients with "weights" in "weighted sums." We now pick up this thread by considering an eye with not one but two aberrations: regular astigmatism which happens to have major axes at 90 and 180 degrees, and coma in the horizontal meridian. For the sake of illustration we also assume that the astigmatism coefficient, C_2^{-2}, turns out to have a value of 0.6 microns, while the coma coefficient, C_3^1, turns out to have a value of 0.2 microns; all others are assumed to be zero. These values indicate fairly high astigmatism and some coma. I.e., in this case the astigmatism is "weightier." Of course we have not yet covered how the values of these coefficients are established, but we know that the capacity of a coefficient to quantify the relative contribution of a Zernike mode requires normalization of that mode.

135.   At this juncture we must reintroduce the *wavefront aberration function*. In spherical polar coordinates—which we used in the past several paragraphs—this function is commonly labeled as

$$W(\rho,\theta),$$

though we relied on Cartesian coordinates to build ("reconstruct") this term in paragraph 43.

136.   The wavefront aberration function leads to the quantification of *the total optical aberration of this eye*, which mathematically appears as a weighted sum based on the constituent aberrations. This means *that the wavefront aberration function is the weighted sum of Zernike polynomials*. Here is the general weighted-sum equation, which is fundamental in the Zernike system:

$$W(\rho,\theta) = \sum_{n,m} C_n^m Z_n^m (\rho,\theta).$$

137.   Spelled out, this equation states that the wavefront at every location in spherical polar coordinates (ρ,θ) is a sum $\sum_{n,m}$ of all Zernike polynomials Z_n^m, weighted by the coefficients C_n^m. The ultimate use of this equation devolves upon solving it for the coefficient C_n^m for every Z_n^m which is present in the eye in question, thus giving us *the magnitude and identity of each aberration*.

The above equation is solved on a unit circle (paragraph 22; this is why spherical polar coordinates are preferred here), presuming that the polynomials are orthogonal. We can also add that all Zernike polynomials together form a "complete set," though this detail is not essential for us; it means that the inventory of all Zernike polynomials exhausts all possibilities.

138.   For just the two aberrations which we devised in paragraph 134, the above equation is

$$W(\rho,\theta) = C_2^{-2}\, Z_2^{-2}\, (\rho,\theta) + C_3^1\, Z_3^1\, (\rho,\theta).$$

Clearly, the refractive status of this eye is composed of only two aberrations. One aberration is described by the Zernike polynomial Z_2^{-2} , which is astigmatism whose wavefront has a shape given by $\sqrt{6}\,\rho^2 \sin 2\,\theta$. (We note no normalization constant here.) We assumed that the "weight" of this Zernike polynomial is 0.6 microns, which is expressed in the value of C_2^{-2} in the above equation. *This value is the contribution of Z_2^{-2} to the overall aberration, to the overall wavefront, and to the wavefront aberration function.*

139.   The other Zernike polynomial in this case, labeled Z_3^1 , is for coma whose individual wavefront has a shape given by $\sqrt{8}\,(3\,\rho^2 - 2)\,\rho \cos\theta$. *Its contribution is 0.2 microns, as expressed in the value of* C_3^1 .

140.   When a wavefront aberration function is written as a weighed sum of Zernike polynomials (here a good synonym is "Zernike basis functions"), the result is a "Zernike expansion." Its gist in this example is the term

$$C_2^{-2}\, Z_2^{-2} + C_3^1\, Z_3^1$$

which here means "0.6 units of astigmatism plus 0.2 units of coma."

Clearly, the wavefront aberration function has been "expanded" or "decomposed" (analyzed) into its constituent weighted aberrations. In this context we continue to use the word "constituent" to indicate those aberrations—those Zernike polynomials—which play a role in the overall wavefront of this eye. That is to say, in this example the optics of the eye suffer from two constituent simultaneous defects.

Of course here we only presumed a rather unusual two-component refractive error and its magnitudes, one which would be rarely encountered in practice. Let us see how we determine these data "in real life."

IDENTIFICATION and QUANTIFICATION of POLYNOMIALS

141. Two critical mathematical questions were posed in paragraph 60: We can now reconsider these more precisely. First, how do we tell—how does our equipment determine—which Zernike basis functions appear in a measured wavefront? That is to say, how do we know which Zernike polynomials are represented in the patient's overall optical status? How do we identify the constituent aberrations?

The second question is, once we identify the constituent Zernike polynomials, how do we find their magnitudes? I.e., how do we determine the values of the corresponding coefficients?

142. This issue is easier to examine in Cartesian coordinates, x and y, while using the example in the previous section. Given the raw data obtained by the H-S sensor for the eye in this instance, *how do we know that the Zernike constituent polynomials are* Z_2^{-2} *and* Z_3^1*, and how do we know the values of* C_2^{-2} *and* C_3^1 . In general then, how do we satisfy the all-inclusive equation

$$W(x,y) = \sum_{n,m} C_n^m Z_n^m (x,y)$$

and satisfy the specific equation for this case,

$$W(x,y) = C_2^{-2} \ Z_2^{-2} \ (x,y) + C_3^1 \ Z_3^1 \ (x,y) ?$$

In the latter "specific" equation, the polynomials and their coefficient are fully labeled.

143. Another way to state the problem is as follows: *What combination of constituent Zernike polynomials and their coefficients fits best into the available wavefront raw data?* This wording implies Zernike analysis, and it suggests the following analogy. The "raw data" tell us we have a total of 10 dollars. This sum is made of coins, including quarters and one-dollar coins. What combination of constituent coins and their quantities fits best into the total? We may even imagine that the "raw data" include the shape of the pile of coins if arranged in stacks of each denomination. Armed with all this information, a unique answer can be obtained. For example, the pile is 9 one-dollar coins and 4 quarters. Then our "coefficients" are 9 and 4, while the "polynomials" are dollar-coins and quarters.

144. The analogy with coins covers a feature we neglected so far. If we so wished, the answer should include, say, dimes and nickels but no pennies. This illustrates that we can decide which kinds of Zernike polynomials are to be sought. For example if our laser is not sufficiently sophisticated to accept "pennies," or if clinical factors so indicate, we can direct the program to "look" no further than a certain order, which means that it will seek to identify and quantify only certain polynomials. Similarly, we can direct the program to report only high-order aberrations and ignore low orders. The mathematical side to making these selections is that in effect we specify the values for n and m to be included, or the highest index to be included if the system accepts the single-index method of naming Zernike polynomials.

◆

145. We are ready for details on Zernike analysis. There are several methods, but we only need an outline of a common approach. As a preview, the main steps are these:

1. We obtain the raw data consisting of displacements, and we convert these data into a collection of slopes. The slopes are used to reconstruct the wavefront.

2. We use the Zernike polynomials in the form of their partial differentials.

3. We place our slopes and our partial differentials into two separate matrices, and then we obtain a dot product. (These terms are explained as we go along.) We note that even though we have obtained the wavefront, we reach back to an earlier stage—our slopes—in order to begin Zernike analysis. This is the overlap mentioned in paragraph 63.

4. The new matrix is subjected to a "best-fit least-square" method for establishing which polynomials and which coefficients fit the data.

5. The constituent Zernike polynomials are identified by their indices and their associated coefficients. Analysis has been accomplished.

6. These results are presented to us for clinical application.

Though the next section, dealing with the mathematical steps in the best-fit least-square method, may be of little interest to some readers (if so please skip to paragraph 164), here are some more details.

146. Having obtained ("reconstructed") $W(x,y)$ from the raw data, we use the concept that the wavefront can be analyzed ("decomposed") into a weighted sum of constituent Zernike polynomials according to the equation from paragraph 136. However, it is easier to use single-index enumeration by the number j (and Cartesian coordinates). Thus our key general equation becomes

$$W(x,y) = \sum_j C_j Z_j(x,y).$$

Though not obvious, we have obtained the overall shape of wavefront for an eye, and now we ask which constituent shapes are represented, as well as how much of each is represented.

147. To continue, we take the first partial derivative of the above equation. (We recall that a derivative [differential] calculates the change in a quantity, and when two variables change independently, the differentials are partial.) This step converts the left side of the above equation back into local slopes or gradients, and it converts the right side to the partial derivatives of the Zernike polynomials. Thus the following equation tells us how the wavefront changes in relation to how the polynomials change, location by location in two dimensions.

$$\frac{\partial W(x,y)}{\partial(x \text{ or } y)} = \sum_j C_j \frac{\partial Z_j(x,y)}{\partial(x \text{ or } y)}$$

We also recall that the local slopes can be calculated from the displacements according to

$$\frac{\Delta(x\ or\ y)}{f} = S \ .$$

148. Therefore,

$$\frac{\partial W(x,y)}{\partial x} = \frac{\Delta x}{f} \quad \text{and} \quad \frac{\partial W(x,y)}{\partial y} = \frac{\Delta y}{f} \ .$$

We see that *the slope at any location on the wavefront has a direct connection to the raw data collected in the form of displacements.* (Paragraphs 42 and 43.)

149. The main parts of the above two equations can be treated as components of vectors or as components of matrices. In this context a vector is a list of components which enumerate or represent all elements of a certain kind of quantity. A matrix is a rectangular table with rows and columns that hold such elements. A dot product (a.k.a. an inner or scalar product) is a special form of multiplication of vectors and matrices. We now lay out the first of two vector/matrix equations.

150. For the first of these, the data for the *slopes* constitutes a column vector "S" which is a vertical list of $\frac{\Delta x}{f}$ and $\frac{\Delta y}{f}$ terms. The number of components is twice the number of spots, since the displacement of each spot is measured horizontally as well as vertically (two-dimensionally).

151. Another column vector, "C," lists the Zernike coefficients. The number of components here is the maximum number of polynomials we elected to consider. Since we are using the single index method of enumerating these, the column has j components. *This column—that is to say, the value of each coefficient—is our "unknown."* (Unknown in the algebraic sense.)

152. As for the matrix which can be called "A," it holds the partial derivatives (partial differentials) of the Zernike polynomials, as in the right side of the partial differential equation in paragraph 147. It has as many rows as vector S, twice the number of spots. It has as many columns as the number of polynomials to be included, which is j. This kind of matrix is called the interaction matrix, though a better name is the gradient matrix. The piston polynomial is not represented. (In theory, the matrix could be infinitely wide, since the number of polynomials can be infinite.)

153. We now have three vectors, S, C, and A. Since the partial differential equation in paragraph 147 sets the pattern, we could write $S = CA$, but the usual arrangement is

$$S = AC \ .$$

Different authors use different labels for these vectors and this matrix, so that cross-comparisons can be confusing. Using our system, we can write an intermediate scheme,

Vector S. Raw data list of $\dfrac{\Delta's}{f}$	=	Interaction matrix A. Column and row list of the partial derivatives of polynomials	Vector C. List of Coefficients C_i

The process of multiplying the vector with data (S) by a matrix to yield the vector with coefficients (C) is also a kind of numerical integration, which in turn is an approximation-type of integration.

154. The problem with the above scheme, i.e., with the equation $S = AC$, is twofold. First, the "unknown" is C, so this equation should be solvable for C. However, it isn't because it represents vector/matrix special (dot) multiplication. Second, we must still find the best-fitting Zernike polynomials for the wavefront data. I.e., we must identify the modes present in this case, while the possibilities are virtually endless. The solutions to these questions are accessible through the process of *least-square fitting*.

155. The general principle of least squares can be illustrated on a "straight curve," i.e., a potentially curved line which now happens to be straight, because this principle can be extended to more complicated functions such as polynomials. We imagine a scatter graph which plots intraocular pressure against age, and viewed from afar, the data points suggest a trend toward higher pressure in advancing age. We sketch a straight line freehand, one that seems to match this trend. Of course some data points fall above our estimated line and others fall below it, and in each such case there is a measurable vertical gap between them. Is the line we drew really the "best fit" for the data?

A simple test would be to see if all the gaps above the line add up to the total of all the gaps below it; this is a "sum of residuals" estimate. However, there are more sophisticated methods (with sub-varieties) which require that each gap be the side of a square. Then the "best-fitting" line is the one that yields the smallest sum of these squares. If the best-fitting line we seek is not straight but curved and sinusoidal, a more complicated multi-parameter procedure is needed, but the goal and principle are the same: to ascertain which line best fits the data. In this case *the outcome consists of a set of polynomials which best fit the measured wavefront.* This is our immediate objective.

Another way to envision how a system can find the best fit is to "let it try" low-order aberrations (simple but likely polynomials) first. Those which fit the raw data are subtracted from the data, and the remaining "residual" becomes the new raw data. Progressively higher order aberrations are "tried" on this residual data, and the process is repeated until the residual is negligible. (Of course this may entail a huge number of "tries," but computerization eases the process.) Finally we tally which aberrations have fit.

156. We can summarize all this quite compactly. Starting with $S = AC$, the goal of best-fitting is to find the *minimum* $\|S - AC\|^2$, i.e., the least square of the absolute difference between S and AC. In fact once you say it, the idea is not as difficult as it seems. We seek the least possible incongruity or discrepancy between the measured data, represented by S, and the available weighted polynomials, represented by AC. Worded in reverse, *we seek the best match between (1) what we measured and (2) the possible weighted polynomials in our inventory.*

157. As an outcome of the least-square search using vector/matrix methods, two matrix-algebra steps arise. One is using the "transposed" matrix of A. The other is using the "inverse" of matrices. The former is indicated by the superscript T. The latter is indicated by the superscript -1. (If matrix A is

a	b
c	d

then its transpose A^T is

a	c
b	d

and the inverse of A is such that

$$AA^{-1} = 1 \ .)$$

158. The result is a new matrix, the "reconstructor" matrix, "R." It turns out that

$$R = (A^T A)^{-1} A^T .$$

Now another vector/matrix scheme can be written, and it is represented by an equation solvable (!) for the unknown coefficient, in which the non-zero coefficients are associated with the best-fitting polynomials. In other words, if a coefficient has a non-zero value, then its associated polynomial—the one with the same index—is present. Thus,

$$SR = C_{best\ fit} \ .$$

These C's identify and quantify the polynomials which are present in this wavefront.

159. Incidentally, this process involves the "root mean square (RMS) error," while RMS depends on the variance. In the use of the least-square method, those coefficients for each polynomial which minimize the variance are identified. Hence we will read the somewhat unclear statement that the root mean square error is minimized. A better assertion is that the least-square method identifies coefficients in a way in which RMS is as small as possible, finding the most mathematically economical selection of polynomials. (Though the analogy is not perfect here, think of preferring \$1.25 in the form of a Dollar bill and a quarter coin rather than in many quarters, dimes, nickels and pennies.) More about variance and RMS shortly.

160. Now we can modify the scheme which we devised in paragraph 43 and which read

"Displacements of spots $\rightarrow$ Slopes $\rightarrow$ Wavefront errors $\rightarrow$ Shape of wavefront."

We can show the role and outcome of least-square fitting during analysis of the wavefront in an enlarged scheme :

Displacements of spots $\rightarrow$ Slopes $\rightarrow$ Wavefront errors $\rightarrow$ Shape of wavefront

Least-square fitting of slopes to derivatives of Zernike polynomials

List of Zernike polynomials weighted by coefficients, which represent the aberrations in this eye.

161. We note that in the latter scheme, Zernike analysis starts as a branch in the reconstruction of the wavefront. In other words we use raw data before they are converted into a wavefront. This is why the terminology (reconstruction vs. analysis) tends to be unclear; see paragraph 199 for a preview of a discussion of the terminology. We also note the importance of indices; *the constituent polynomials and their quantifying coefficients can be succinctly labeled and listed by their indices.*

162. Clearly, the ascertaining of a best fit is a crucial facet in analyzing the measured wavefront. This process converts a set of displacement measurements into its constituent aberrations (in the form of certain Zernike polynomials) and it reveals how much of each aberration (in the form of a coefficient) is present in this wavefront. Incidentally, best-fit searches also underpin most Fourier systems.

163. Obviously the steps outlined above are complex. For even more detail, Maeda clearly shows one way and Tolstoba another (see Bibliography). One of the directions of basic research in this area is finding alternatives; for example see the two articles by Zavyalona et al. and the article by Shiode et al.

164. In any case, the end-product is a list of "weighed Zernike polynomials," which is a set of coefficient-and-polynomial units, as we mentioned in paragraph 61. This set forms an "expansion" or "series." Each unit is a "Zernike prescription," and it is the wavefront counterpart of spectacle Rx: *how much* and *which kind* of aberrations the patient has. In essence then, the equation

$$W(x,y) = \sum_j C_j Z_j(x,y)$$

has been solved. (This equation still employs the single-index method for identifying coefficients and polynomials; shortly we will revert to the double-index method.) At the same time we have the information needed to produce a map or model or other descriptions of the wavefront, which means that we "know" the wavefront and what it contains. Of course the ultimate goal is to let our laser "know" what to do. (Paragraph 9.)

165. We note that although the wavefront is a potentially very complicated three-dimensional structure, we have deduced its shape from two-dimensional measurements on a reference plane. While our ability to do so is interesting, our ability to extract the identity of Zernike polynomials and their coefficients out of the same data is a very useful accomplishment of applied mathematics. (It adds to my gratification in majoring in math despite my advisors' advice in the 1950's that this was a waste for pre-med students.)

166. An important warning needs to be stated here. As sophisticated the procedure for ascertaining coefficients appears to be, the size of the pupil is very important. Indeed aberrometry may reveal a very different set of polynomials and coefficients for the same eye with a different pupil size. In general, more aberrations and more severity of aberrations are found under mydriasis. We will return to this fact because it also applies to other optical assessments.

167. At this point let us review the following helpful features of Zernike polynomials:

1. They are orthogonal (mathematically independent) over a unit circle.

2. Their average or mean is zero.

3. They have unit variance.

168. These mathematical characteristics provide the ability to compare contributions by different Zernike polynomials against the overall wavefront, which is a weighted sum. That is to say, these stipulations, based on forms of normalization, are essential to the successful participation of all polynomials in handling the total aberration. In particular, the best-fitting procedure would be far more complicated if the Zernike polynomials were not orthogonal. The best-fit principle works well because the coefficient of each can accurately reveal the amount of the corresponding aberration in the weighted total regardless of which or how many other coefficients and aberrations are involved. Otherwise, the presence of one Zernike polynomial would alter and disturb the coefficients of others.

VARIANCE and RMS

169.   It is time for a more accurate definition and discussion of variance. (See paragraph 68.) To minimize confusion in an already confusing topic, a few basic concepts are important.

Variance is a statistical term used to show the spread of a distribution of values, but it is best that we set aside the general statistical application of variance. In our context, variance provides an assessment of the severity of the total aberration present in an amertopic eye; in short, it tells us "how bad" the optics are and roughly "how bad" the eyesight could be. Another way of thinking about this is to ask how hilly and uneven is the surface of the wavefront. Variance provides this information by indicating *how far weighted polynomials (the wavefront errors) are from their average.* A further assessment of the status of an eye is afforded by the RMS which, as we will see, is based on variance.

At this point we must make a clear distinction. *Each weighted polynomial* has its own variance. I.e., each coefficient-and-its-polynomial unit—each *CZ* unit or each Zernike prescription—can deviate from the average of all units for this eye. However, the *overall wavefront* also has a variance, and this *total variance is a sum of its constituent variances.* (This is possible since all Zernike polynomials and all *CZ* units are independent of each other.)

The logical way an individual variance—the variance for one weighted polynomial—can be calculated is in two steps. First, we can calculate of how far from an average it is. This means subtracting the average from a coefficient-and-polynomial unit; i.e., calculating the value of $(CZ) - (\text{Average } CZ)$.

Second, since this result can be a negative number, we square the result so the outcome is always positive; this gives $(CZ - \text{Average } CZ)^2$, which is $(C - \text{Average } C)^2$ for every case. Meanwhile, we ensured zero average for each polynomial (paragraphs 104-106); in short, each Average $C = 0$. Therefore the term $(C - \text{Average } C)^2$ becomes simply C^2, and an individual variance is simply C^2. Since the value is also squared, variance may be magnified and is always positive. (In emmetropia it is zero.) The standard label for variance in statistics is σ^2, but for clarity I prefer "*Var*."

We can express the same conclusion in words alone. Coefficients represent the severity of aberrations, so their variance is critical. Variance of a coefficient is its deviation from an average. Squaring what remains rectifies the variance but can magnify it.

170.   In short, *the variance of each weighted polynomial* is such that

$$Var_{each} = C^2.$$

Later we will use this equation as an example. More importantly now, the variance of the overall wavefront—the *total variance*—is the *sum* of the square of *every* coefficient in play. In equation form, and including the standard indices,

$$Var_{TOTAL} = \sum_{n,m}(C_n^m)^2.$$

Clearly, each mode found in an eye imparts its variance upon the total variance, and a relatively large individual C accounts for a relatively very large portion of the total variance. We also recall that in the best-fit least-square method, the resulting coefficients are those which minimize the variance; more on this point shortly.

171. Armed with the double-index method of listing Zernike polynomials, we can now also give the mathematical criterion of *unit variance* for a Zernike system: The variance of Z_n^m is 1 for all values of m and n. Also see Note 5 on page 89.

◆

172. We are ready for the RMS, the root mean square, also called the RMS error. In addition to considering the number and magnitudes of the various coefficients, we need a way of assessing the quality of the overall wavefront, including some way of assessing the contribution of low- and high-order modes. This information is provided by the RMS values. We define RMS as *the square root of the total variance*, which in turn is the sum of the squared coefficients (as above in paragraphs 169 and 170). In equation form,

$$RMS = \sqrt{Total\ Variance} = \sqrt{\sum_{n,m} C_n^{m^2}} \ .$$

This means that coefficients can be negative, but—like the variance—the RMS can only be positive (or zero). Like coefficients, the units for RMS are microns.

Before going further we note that calculating an RMS is unnecessary if the entire refractive error can be quantified by only one coefficient and one mode. In other words, RMS's are of value only when the wavefront is deformed by multiple aberrations. This is obvious from the above equation; if the sum, $\sum$, is made up of only one coefficient (one C), then the square root of its square is that coefficient, except it is always positive. ($\sqrt{C^2} = C$.)

173. Incidentally, we implied that RMS in our setting is analogous to the standard deviation in statistics. We say that the RMS is akin to the standard deviation of the slope of the wavefront. Statisticians may point out that standard deviation is the square root of the variance, which is the *mean* of the summed squares of the coefficients, but since our coefficients are normalized, we are allowed to use RMS as we have defined it.

174. Normalization to unit variance means that each higher-order Zernike polynomial tends to minimize the RMS. This notion is tied to the use of least squares to find the best-fitting polynomials. After each fit, the RMS error is minimized, and in this way a progressively better set of polynomials is identified; we recall paragraph 159. (The point that each polynomial tends to minimize the RMS is useful, because then the addition of lower-order aberrations can only raise the RMS. On the other hand there is automatic compensation in Zernike polynomials such that additional aberrations in one order minimize the RMS, lest the RMS would be exaggerated.)

175. The primary clinical advantage of the RMS is that it hinges directly on the variance, while variance in the wavefront is the main determinant of the quality of the image of which the eye is capable. We can think of RMS as a more sophisticated form of variance and as a better gauge of "wavefront quality." While the RMS pools the effects of many coefficients, it is independent of which aberrations are constituents of the overall wavefront in this case.

176. When the RMS is presented clinically, it is usually broken down into three amounts:

1. the total RMS,

2. the proportion of low-order RMS,

3. and the proportion of high-order RMS.

These amounts lend themselves to bar graphs, though such presentation is generally unnecessary.

177. Normally, an emmetropic eye has an RMS <0.20 microns—ideally its RMS is zero—but as we will see this depends on pupil size. Most eyes that come to routine refractive surgery have less that 0.4 microns of high-order RMS, and an excessive pre-operative high-order RMS value means that an ideal surgical result may be difficult to achieve.

178. RMS is not perfect; for example some aberrations, notably high-order astigmatism and coma, can cause very poor visual acuity even when the RMS is low. Moreover, the size of the pupil is significant; the bigger it is the more accurate is an RMS, and in general RMS is higher during mydriasis. Conversely, a small pupil may hide high-order aberrations, and it may suppress the RMS.

A dramatic use of all three amounts in paragraph 176 might be in a patient with apparently normal anatomy who has near-plano optics based on traditional refraction, who complains of poor vision, and who has demonstrably poor image quality. We might find minimal low-order RMS but sizable high-order RMS. A few years ago we might have ascribed this paradox to "irregular astigmatism" and resorted to some kind of contact lens. Today, armed with any kind of wavefront-guided refractive surgery, we can make a more accurate diagnosis and consider more direct treatment.

179. Incidentally, this kind of situation—very mild low-order aberrations and low-order RMS but significant high-order aberrations and high-order RMS—unfortunately may arise *after* refractive surgery (and of course it may account for patient dissatisfaction despite a near-plano post-operative refraction). Some problems are easy to trace. For example inadvertent decentration of ablation can induce coma, and cyclotorsion can aggravate astigmatism.

Other problems are more subtle, such as the induction of spherical aberration. While the exact mechanism is unclear, this complication is an unintended increase in the natural oblateness of the cornea (which normally attenuates spherical aberration). To make matters worse, pre-existing spherical aberration may be associated with over-correction of pre-op myopia—the spherical equivalent shifts forward—which may account for excessive low-order RMS. In any case the separation of RMS's into low-order and high-order is very useful; examples come later.

ASTIGMATISM *in the* ZERNIKE SYSTEM

180. We turn to how astigmatism is handled in the Zernike system, which is doubly important since the other "meridional" aberrations—those which have axes or angular orientations—are handled similarly. The latter include tilt, coma, and complicated astigmatism. However, obviously simple regular astigmatism is the representative instance on which we should focus (pun intended).

The basic idea is that when we superimpose two astigmatic lenses, a new astigmatic unit is created with a new Rx. Likewise a simple astigmatic aberration can be decomposed into two weighted constituent aberrations. *These can be described by the two Zernike polynomials for astigmatism.* In essence, such two polynomials—which reside in the same order but have opposite-signed meridional frequencies—behave like two apposed Jackson cross-cylinders in that they are resolved into one astigmatic Rx, depending on their powers and the angle between them.

181. As we said, the other meridional aberrations follow similar patterns: Their description requires a pair of polynomials which share an order but have opposite frequencies. We can think of such pairs as descriptions of one aberration, but each member of the pair is oriented along a different axis.

In each case a weighted blend of certain polynomials determines the resultant orientation and magnitude. For example, coma oriented along a certain oblique axis is described by a blend of the two polynomials which describe the same coma (and tilt, which go together) but which differ in orientation in space. Mathematically this difference is easy to recognize. Each row of the pyramid in paragraph 130 has pairs of Zernike polynomials which differ with respect to the sign of the meridional frequency index in the two-index notation.

182. Here are some details about regular astigmatism, though these include defocus, as we will see: The Zernike polynomial Z_2^{-2} describes oblique astigmatism with the major axes at 45 and 135 degrees. The Zernike polynomial Z_2^2 describes with-the-rule astigmatism at 90 and 180 degrees; both appear in the third row in the pyramid in paragraph 130, sharing one order but having frequencies of opposite sign. (One of these is a sine and the other a cosine.) *By blending these in proper amounts of each—with proper coefficients for each—any axis and power can be represented.*

Incidentally, meridional aberrations are said to be symmetric (a mirror image is identical) or asymmetric, though the complete term, spherically asymmetric, is more descriptive. Examples of the latter are coma and trefoil, to which we will return. A quick way to tell is that if the order is even (second, fourth), the aberration is symmetric.

183. Since defocus (myopia and hyperopia) and simple astigmatism share the same Zernike order, an obvious question is how an ordinary *sphero-cylindrical error* is described in this system. The answer is through a combination of these three modes and their coefficients in a specific proportion.

We note that the second Zernike order includes Z_2^{-2} and Z_2^2 for astigmatism as well as Z_2^0 for defocus, which has a frequency of zero. The last of these represents defocus only, which implies that the Zernike system treats pure myopia and hyperopia as "spherical astigmatism." In this sense, defocus is simply "astigmatism without an axis."

184. We might expect the sign of the defocus coefficient C_2^0 (which is the coefficient for the Zernike polynomial Z_2^0) to be negative when the spherical part of the prescription is myopia and positive in hyperopia. However, the correlation is not necessarily logical. Indeed, depending on the convention used, we often find myopia described by a positive coefficient and hyperopia by a negative coefficient. Of course no matter what its +/− sign, C_2^0 is a function of the amount of myopia or hyperopia. (The Zernike polynomial for myopia describes a wavefront with a concave shape, and Zernike polynomials for myopia and astigmatism describe a wavefront that has a concave warped shape. See also Note 2 on page 89.)

185. Even for just regular astigmatism without defocus, the computational particulars are complicated. The amount of astigmatism depends on a ratio of the squares of C_2^{-2} and C_2^2, which of course describe the amount of 45/135 degree astigmatism and 90/180 degree astigmatism respectively. That ratio is $\dfrac{(C_2^{-2})^2 - (C_2^2)^2}{\sqrt{(C_2^{-2})^2 + (C_2^2)^2}}$. (Astigmatism is "high" when one of these C's is large and the other small. The algebraic sign of the ratio indicates mainly "with the rule" vs. mainly "against the rule" astigmatism.) The exact axis of astigmatism is calculated from another ratio, proportional to $\dfrac{1}{\tan}\left(\dfrac{-C_2^{-2}}{C_2^2}\right)$. We note that this arrangement is quite parsimonious in the sense that the blend of only two numbers, C_2^{-2} and C_2^2, suffices to pin down both the axis and amount. (Navigators and aviators may be aware that these computations are issues in vector resolution.)

186. Incidentally, in the context of blended polynomials, another way to index Zernike polynomials and coefficients is to combine meridional pairs and to specify the axis. For example a combination of C_2^{-2} and C_2^2 can be combined into "C_{22} at 60 degrees." In this system, one blended coefficient suffices, but then spelling out the axis is essential. We encounter this indexing method only occasionally in the literature, though it echoes the way we commonly describe astigmatism. For instance "C_{22} at 60 degrees" might mean "three diopters at 60 degrees."

187. Many aberrations do not have what we routinely call an axis or an angular direction, but they have an "up" and a "down," or a "left" and "right," or a "vertical" and "horizontal." The best example here is coma. The polynomial Z_3^{-1} and coefficient C_3^{-1} describe vertical coma. This defect consists of a "bulge" in one half of the wavefront and a depression in the other, but the obvious question is which one—bulge or depression—is in the upper half. This difference appears in the algebraic sign of the coefficient. If the bulge is "up," then C_3^{-1} is positive, and if the depression is "up," C_3^{-1} is negative. The same convention applies to tilt; the algebraic sign indicates which way the tilt faces.

We see that some pairs of meridional polynomials are 90 degrees apart, such as tilt and coma, while others are 45 degrees apart, such as ordinary stigmatism.

188. Given this peculiar approach to axes and orientations, let us compare how we clinicians refract, versus how "Zernike polynomials refract." Manual refraction essentially includes determining a sphere and selecting a cylinder power while rotating its axis. We could do this "the Zernike way" instead. We select two Jackson cross-cylinders and add them together until the resolved axis and power are satisfactory. When we get to the Fourier system, we will see more ways in which this contrast in methodology is significant.

◆

189. At several junctures we saw groupings of Zernike polynomials, while these associations at first glance may not have made sense. For example, in paragraph 130, fourth row, *why should coma and trefoil be juxtaposed?* Of course their common subscript, 3, suggests they share the third order, but that does not tell us enough. How are coma and trefoil linked at all? For a hint, let us recall how regular astigmatism is handled, namely by the judicious addition of two polynomials.

With regard to trefoil and coma, we must recognize three details, even if these are difficult to envision: First, trefoil is like ordinary astigmatism but it has three major axes rather than two. Second, and more to the point, the location of maximum wavefront error can be eccentric; it can be shifted away from the visual axis in a certain direction, as is more obvious with coma (think also of keratoconus). Third, the amount of the maximum error is also significant. As mentioned, aberrations of this kind are said to be "asymmetric" or, better yet, "spherically asymmetric."

The purpose of the two coma polynomials in this setting is to accommodate eccentricity in trefoil. This arrangement works as follows. An eye has trefoil, the maximum point of which is off center by a certain amount in a certain direction. (Imagine that the surface of Alaska has a trefoil shape, but Mt. McKinley is not in the center.) By including a judicious combination of two coma polynomials, the system can depict this trefoil even though it is decentered. In effect, *eccentric trefoil is trefoil plus coma.* Hence this group contains polynomials for trefoil as well as for coma. On the one hand, such arrangements are ingenious solutions to the problem of describing various very complex refractive errors. On the other hand, they make for intricate mathematics.

CLINICAL OUTPUT

190.   Let us say that our H-S device has done its work, and that all the Zernike polynomial data have been processed. What clinically useful or interesting information becomes available? The following items are customarily presented in one or another format (and Fourier-based systems provide very similar outputs):

1.   A model and/or map of the wavefront, along with its interpretation.

2.   A listing of aberrations, often in the form of a bar graph, showing which ones were found in this eye, together with the magnitudes of these aberrations.

3.   RMS values for low, high, and total orders.

4.   Estimates of image quality, usually including PSF, MTF, and/or the Strehl ratio.

The above list in not exhaustive, and it omits critical information from other diagnostic sources such as pupil size, manual refraction, keratometry, topography, corneal thickness, etc. However, the latter data do not depend on Zernike polynomials.

Let us comment on the four items enumerated above and include definitions of the terms.

191.   Three-dimensional models, maps, and diagrams of wavefronts are usually colored to show depth. They appear in nearly all scientific and promotional literature—including "info-mercials"—dealing with this topic. We should keep in mind that such renditions depict the "mountainous terrain" of the wavefront and represent collections of "altitudes" out of which a model, map, or diagram is created.

(Another measure occasionally reported is peak-to-valley differences, which in a sense justifies the analogy with altitudes and mountains, but it does not reveal how much of the entire wavefront surface is abnormal, only the maximum extent of the abnormality.)

Since wavefronts represent refractive errors, an aberrometer can also provide an Rx, as does manual refraction. Of course a major discrepancy between the Rx generated by the aberrometer and the Rx obtained clinically should be a "red flag" suggesting consequential pathology.

192.   Generally our equipment can handle at most 10 Zernike orders, which means about 60 aberrations, though anything over 6 orders may be superfluous. Presenting these and their coefficients as bar graphs is logical and easy. The polynomials that were found are usually listed on the horizontal axis, commonly using the single-index method, and the vertical height of each coefficient represents its magnitude, commonly in microns. The index itself lets us name the aberrations; for example we know which index stands for defocus, astigmatism, etc.

(The coefficients can be positive, negative or zero. We recall that the positivity or negativity of any coefficient may depend on the axis or orientation; for example a cornea with a superior ectasia may have a positive coefficient and one with an inferior ectasia may have a negative coefficient, though this custom is arbitrary.)

Here is an example of a bar graph:

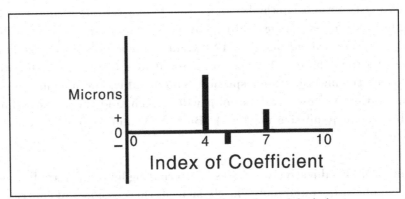

Bar graph showing the coefficients of three polynomials, index
numbers 4, 5 and 7. Their magnitudes appear in microns. Coefficients
can be negative (coefficient 5 in this example). We know which
aberrations are present from the indices.

193.   We already discussed RMS's in principle, but now let us calculate the total RMS, the
low-order RMS and the high-order RMS for an imaginary case. Of course the reason to isolate
low-order and high-order aberrations is that each has special diagnostic meanings. For example
high-order defects can obscure critical low-order defects, particularly on a map or diagram of
the wavefront.

For simplicity we again assume that only two refractive errors are present: 0.6 microns of
45/135 degree regular astigmatism and 0.2 microns of horizontal coma.

First we need the individual variances, each of which is the sum of the square of the coefficient
(as in paragraph 170). The square of 0.6 is 0.36. The square of 0.2 is 0.04.

The total variance is therefore 0.36 + 0.04 or 0.40. (Again, the entire variance of an eye is the
sum of all its component variances, while each Zernike polynomial is independent. Thus, each
Zernike polynomial can contribute its weighed share to the overall wavefront.)

The total RMS, here the square root of the total variance 0.40, is about 0.63, suggesting
significant ametropia.

The low-order coefficient (there is only one in this example) is 0.6. Its square is 0.36, and the
square root of 0.36 is 0.6, which is the low-order RMS, suggesting that most of the ametropia
is low-order.

The high-order coefficient (there is only one in this example) is 0.2. Its square is 0.04, and the
square root of 0.04 is 0.2, which is the high-order RMS. This value suggests that very little of
the ametropia is high-order.

60

194. Zernike polynomials are quite effective in describing wavefronts—though we will discuss some limitation—but they do not provide a quantification of the quality of the image when aberrations exist. Various methods can be used to express *image quality*. Of course total variance ultimately determines image quality, but we have more specific ways. Two commonly used criteria are the *point spread function* (PSF) and the *modulation transfer function* (MTF). The former, in short, estimates the blur of a point-like image, and the word "spread" adequately describes the meaning; some spread is unavoidable, and of course less is better. In effect, the former estimates how clearly a point will be seen, and the latter estimates contrast resolution. (Here again pupil size matters.) Both PSF and MTF can be calculated from Zernike polynomials.

195. To obtain an MTF subjectively, a series of alternating light and dark lines are presented, and as these are made thinner and more closely spaced, there is a loss of contrast. That loss is expressed in terms of the "frequency" of the lines, which means how closely spaced they are. (The word "frequency" is confusing because in this setting it is a spatial term; pairs of lines per millimeter for example, not per second.)

196. As an example of another quantitative assessment of optical performance, we can calculate the *Strehl ratio*. All optical systems incur a certain amount of diffraction.[9] A circular diffraction pattern—called an Airy disk, which looks like an archery target—has a certain brightness at its center. This intensity of light is reduced at the center and diffused by any aberration. The ratio between the intensity with aberrations and the intensity without aberrations is the Strehl ratio; ideally it is 1.0 or 100% for the emmetropic eye, and anything below 0.8 or 80% correlates with reduced acuity. Another interpretation of the Strehl ratio is the eye's best PSF divided by the aberration-free PSF.

197. We should not confuse PSF, MTF, and similar image functions with RMS, which is a direct measure of the quality of the wavefront.

198. Of course the final step is the *raison d'etre* of the entire effort. The *ablation profile*—also called the ablation target map—is the set of instructions sent to the laser for eradicating the errors in the wavefront. In theory, the ablation profile is designed from the shape of the wavefront, though in mathematical practice it draws on more basic data. Various technical and optical refinements for ablation profiles exist, and these also incorporate data from other sources, such as refraction, corneal topography, pachymetry, etc. The design of ablation profiles, which is a separate and vast topic beyond our scope, naturally is complicated by exactly how laser energy affects corneal tissue and by how the eye heals. Empiric experience-based data plays a major role.

---

[9] In this context diffraction is of great interest in quantum mechanics, as it is evidence of the probabilistic wave-behavior of photons.

FURTHER KEY DEFINITIONS

Since we are "between the two systems," Zernike's and Fourier's, this is an opportunity to discuss some important mathematical items common to both, in part because these are often unclear in the literature. We will define them in simple language now, even at the risk of redundancy, and even though they include Fourier concepts to be covered later. These terms are as follows.

Analysis (Zernike or Fourier)
Deconstruction
Synthesis (Zernike or Fourier)
Domain

199. We recall that a wavefront is reconstructed from the raw data usually provided by a H-S device. To a large extent, reconstruction of a wavefront is similar in both systems, since both can use the same kind of raw data. Once a wavefront has been reconstructed, the polynomials and their coefficients are identified from within that wavefront by means of *analysis*. The bulk of what we call the Zernike or Fourier system is actually Zernike or Fourier analysis. *Analysis yields the constituent weighted polynomials*, and it often applies a best-fit method.

In Zernike systems the wavefront is treated as a *shape* which has constituent shapes; see paragraph 9. In Fourier systems the polynomials are "wavelets," which as we shall see is a crucial concept based in the idea that the wavefront can be treated as a *wave*. To distinguish this wave from a constituent wavelet, at times we call it a "total wave." (Technically, Fourier waves and wavelets are both polynomials, but making the distinction between them facilitates the discussion.)

200. The term analysis is more commonly used as "Fourier analysis"; we hear of Zernike analysis only occasionally, though the latter is a legitimate and useful term. As synonyms for Zernike analysis, we often hear of a "Zernike expansion," since analysis yields a list—an expansion—of weighted polynomials. However, expansions are really the output of analysis. We also hear of "Fourier series," which is equivalent to a "Fourier expansion." Again, the series is the output of analysis. As we will also find in the literature, it is tempting to use the word "decomposition" for "analysis," but if we had to be very meticulous, the former should be used as a synonym for deconstruction of a wavefront back to its raw data.

In any case, let us again make this point explicitly, though we will say more about it in the Fourier context:

Reconstruction from raw data → a wavefront.

Zernike analysis of a wavefront → weighted polynomials within the wavefront treated as a shape.

Fourier analysis of a wavefront → weighted wavelets within the wavefront treated as a wave.

The list of weighted polynomials or weighted wavelets is an expansion or a series. In either case polynomials and wavelets correspond to optical aberrations, and as we indicated, their respective collections found in an eye describe the refractive status.

201. Most of the distinguishing features of the two systems reside in the methods of analysis and, to a lesser extent, in the methods of synthesis. Strictly speaking, Zernike and Fourier analyses are separate processes within their respective systems, though there is overlap with other steps (paragraph 145). Hence many authors take liberties which blur the separations.

202. We can start with a wavefront and *deconstruct* it into slopes and raw data. Deconstruction is a kind of decomposition. We note that this process "runs backwards," from a wavefront to raw data. In strict terminology, it is *not* the same as analysis, which finds constituent weighted polynomials within a wavefront. In this sense, analysis "runs forwards."

203. It is also possible to start with constituent polynomials and coefficients in order to recreate the wavefront. This is *synthesis*, usually part of the term Fourier synthesis, where the starting point is a collection of weighted wavelets and the endpoint is a total wave.

204. Deconstruction and synthesis are often used in research to compare Zernike and Fourier systems. For example we can start with raw data to reconstruct a wavefront, and we analyze this wavefront using both systems.

We then have constituent Zernike polynomials and Fourier wavelets. Next we use the two sets of outcomes to synthesize two wavefronts, one of which of course relied on Zernike data and the other on Fourier data.

We deconstruct each wavefront to retrieve the corresponding raw data. Finally we compare the two sets of raw data to see which comes closer to what we started with. Presumably the "winner" points to the better system. See Note 6 on page 89.

205. Certain additional details about graphs will be important. We can use our diagrams for clarification. In paragraph 235 a curve or wave is graphed in x-y coordinates. The x coordinate or x axis runs running horizontally. Here this axis is marked in degrees and radians, since it represents going around a circle; see paragraphs 73 and 74, where we went around a tower.

The point is that we covered some *distance* (even if we ended up where we began). In almost all graphic presentations, such a distance is represented by an x axis drawn as a straight line, even if it represents a distance that is not straight.

As we progressed along (around) x while measuring heights, a sine curve was generated, shown as a changing amount along the y axis. (This vertical axis is called the "ordinate.") That is to say, a point (on a vertical meter-stick) shifted up and down along y as we moved horizontally along x. Of course then y is also a distance, though in our diagram we call it an amplitude or a coefficient.

206.   An important point is that x and y can represent *other quantities besides distances.* Here y can represent a coefficient, which is a numeral, but it can represent weight, percentage, etc. The x axis could even be distance expressed as speed during a time interval, as in paragraph 237. Moreover the x axis may represent *time* (rather than space), and in fact then the identical sine curve can be generated. Imagine that we walked around our tower in one minute, in which case the measured height changed during that time. Then we could re-label the horizontal axis as t (rather than x).

207.   This point brings us to the concept of a "domain." This general algebraic term has a specific meaning in our setting. When we work with a curve or wave which is graphed or diagramed such that the x axis is time, we say that this curve or wave is in the "time domain," in which it is one-dimensional. When the x axis is distance, we say that this curve or wave is in the "space domain," and then the x can represent more than one dimension. When we set up a graph or diagram with the x axis signifying frequency, as we will do for Fourier analysis, the content of this graph is in the "frequency domain." Finally, other domains are possible, including one which we will call the "index domain."

Thus *the sine curve in the diagram in paragraph 75 is in the space domain, and in general our wavefront diagrams are in the space domain.* We can even say that results of our wavefront reconstructions are routinely *in the space domain.* This means that reconstruction in effect converts refractive errors (aberrations) into wavefronts, but then these are in the space domain, which of course makes sense since as wavefronts are treated as shapes.

In sharp contrast, the graph in paragraph 192 is *not* in the space domain. Although we do not routinely encounter the term in the literature, we can say that this graph is in the "index domain." The point is that Zernike analysis has converted a wavefront which was in the space domain into a graph in another more practical domain, one which describes the optical status of the eye in question.

We stress this notion because we will see that *a Fourier system converts wavefronts in space into an end-product in a frequency domain.* The result is similar to a spectral analysis in that we learn how much of the content of the wavefront lies within various ranges of frequency. On the one hand this detail makes technical comparisons between Fourier and Zernike systems problematic, particularly since it is harder to visualize how clinically useful information can be extracted from data in the form of frequencies. We can however say that in effect Fourier frequencies are analogous to Zernike indices. On the other hand the mathematics of frequency domains is simpler and more versatile. Let us now examine the details.

FOURIER POLYNOMIALS IN OPHTHALMOLOGY

A BIT OF HISTORY and BASIC PRINCIPLES

208.   We have concentrated on the ophthalmologic aspects of Zernike systems, but it is time to turn to their Fourier counterpart. While much of the material covered so far also applies to a typical Fourier system, and while the remaining differences are mainly mathematical, these differences have definite clinical and practical consequences. Again, the distinction between Fourier systems in general and a particular Fourier system is not critical, especially since few manufacturers of LASIK equipment have adopted any Fourier system; Zernike systems are more widely used.

In general, information and references on the ophthalmologic uses of Zernike's mathematics are much easier to locate than for Fourier's methods. For this reason I provide more hard-to-find details and more citations for the latter. (Since a Fourier system is somewhat more unified than Zernike's, the plural term, "Fourier systems," rarely appears in the pertinent literature.)

209.   But first, a bit of history. About a century before Zernike, the mathematician Jean Baptiste (Joseph) Fourier (1768-1830) had centered his efforts on what is now called the Fourier series, though the initial context was the study of conduction of heat through solid masses. Fourier was not concerned with the quality of telescopes, so that his system does not specifically deal with optical defects. Nevertheless this system is quite versatile and addresses the general nature of waves. Meanwhile it turns out that human refractive errors, even very complicated ones, can be treated mathematically as waves, and greater complexity in such waves poses no significant obstacle in their analysis by means of Fourier mathematics. That is to say, a Fourier system can faithfully describe complex aberrations because they are—mathematically speaking—wave-like, and because such a system can handle complex mathematical waves.

210.   As an introduction to Fourier systems, characteristics of the Zernike approach should be emphasized; these reflect the history of optical science, and they will help clarify the main issues. Here are two introductory statements based on these characteristic:

   1) *The critical components of telescopes are circular mirrors and lenses.*

   2) *Telescopes do not get keratoconus.*

211.   Now we retrieve the statement to the effect that the critical components of telescopes are circular. These must be fabricated to very stringent tolerances, and in essence Zernike's mathematics had been designed to assess their quality. Consequently, Zernike polynomials are well suited to a circular wavefront and a circular pupil, and spherical polar coordinates are advantageous. However, most human pupils are not exactly round, which means that any measurements made by a H-S device outside a perfect circle cannot be accepted by Zernike systems.

212.   There is a related issue: In part because a spherical polar system is used in the Zernike system, and in part because of how locations are compared on the reference plane of a H-S device (paragraphs 33, 34, and 35), the measurement of displacements requires a minimum amount of space on that reference plane. This means that the total number of data points—"spots"—available to Zernike analysis is limited, even when the pupil is large. The usual maximum is 40 useable spots, though often fewer. A corollary is that technical faults which interfere with the registration of a spot represents a significant loss of data. Please keep the number 40 in mind, because the Fourier system can accept a much larger number.

213. We note another subtle corollary: Because of the radial structure of a typical Zernike polynomial, the variations are wider near the periphery than at the center. This means that more polynomial terms are needed to describe a defect in the wavefront near the pupillary edge. This in turn means that the system encourages over-sampling at the center, which introduces artifacts. This issue may not arise where a uniform *x-y* Cartesian system can be used. We should keep this fine point in mind also, since certain Fourier algorithms function well in uniform Cartesian systems.

214. Now we invoke the second statement by way of an example. Even if "telescopes do not get keratoconus," telescopes as well as human eyes can be afflicted by coma, wherein half the cornea has a bulge and the other has a concavity. Keratoconus then looks like coma without the concavity. Zernike's system is well equipped to describe coma by means of two simple polynomials, but Zernike had no need to design polynomials for keratoconus.[10] To analyze this defect, his system first treats it like coma, and then it uses additional polynomials to cancel the nonexistent concavity, as we discussed in paragraphs 89 and 90.

These extra polynomials are of a higher order, and one of the issues with Zernike polynomials is that descriptions of high-order errors tend to smooth out subtle features, so that resolution is attenuated. (This smoothing is not always disadvantageous, as we will relate later.) The point is that a description of a simple defect—e.g., one ectasia—ends up invoking a chain of progressively more complex Zernike polynomials, and in the process other features may be obscured.

215. The Fourier system does not react this way to a solitary ectasia. As a preview, the defect is analyzed as a wave which consists of a sum of simple waves ("wavelets"). If many wavelets are needed to describe the initial wave, even to cancel a nonexistent feature, they are all equally simple, and their addition entails no smoothing. (Again, smoothing may sometimes be "a good thing.")

◆

216. We shall now step back and consider Fourier's general ideas. Like Zernike's mathematics, Fourier's is a problem-solving tool, though not specialized to optics. Fourier mathematics is used in many branches of science, economics, sociology, and other medical specialties (e.g., vascular diseases). The application of Fourier's ideas entails numerous steps, procedures, algorithms and protocols, with many ways to execute these. We will confine ourselves mainly to one representative scheme and mention only a few variations and innovations. On the other hand the discussion will cover enough material for readers who skipped the chapters on Zernike.

---

[10] A warp in the mirror of a telescope usually causes one part of the mirror to bulge forward and another to bulge backwards. Such a mirror in effect has coma. It is unlikely for a defective mirror to have the equivalent of keratoconus or an ectasia.

217. The Fourier system, like Zernike's, is based on the "expansions of polynomials." This process in turn is based on the idea that a complicated quantity can be "expanded" or "analyzed" into a series of constituent weighted polynomials, like a whole is the sum of its parts. In Fourier systems, that "whole" is a wave. Accordingly, the fundamental statement in Fourier's system is this:

Any periodic function can be written as a weighted sum of sine and cosine waves of different frequencies. Let us dissect this sentence and explain its terms for our purposes. It contains six parts.

1. A "periodic function" is a *wave*. The key associated concept here is that *the human ocular wavefront can be treated mathematically as a wave.*

2. A "function" is some *numerical relationship* between mathematical variables. A working definition of a function is anything expressible by an equation.

3. "Can be written as" means, in short, "=," though in this context this phrase has an additional connotation which Fourier wished to convey. Please re-read the original statement but replace "can be written as" with "*can be represented by*" or "*is equivalent to*" or—most aptly for us—"*can be reconstructed from.*"

4. A "weighted sum" is the same as in Zernike's system: Each member—each addend—is multiplied by a *coefficient*, one which expresses the mathematical influence of that addend on the sum. More precisely, if an addend happens to represent a discreet aberration—say, defocus—then the coefficient gives its magnitude or amplitude; how much defocus.

5. "Sines and cosines" are trigonometric functions and they are kinds of *waves. These waves are added together in the (weighed) sum.* For identification we call them "*wavelets*," so that their (weighted) sum equals the "*wave.*" A wave is the whole, and constituent wavelets are its parts. If it is not essential to specify whether sine or cosine wavelets are involved, we will use the general term "*sinusoidal*," and such wavelets are simply "*sinusoids.*"

6. These wavelets differ in their "frequency," which has a specific meaning we will discuss shortly. For now let it suffice that *frequency* means *how fast the wavelets repeat.*

The above statement can now be reworded: *Any wave can be reconstructed from a weighted sum of sinusoidal wavelets with different frequencies.*

218. We should detour briefly to amplify points which would have made little sense earlier. We touched on some of these in paragraphs 199-207 because they bridge Zernike and Fourier terms, but they are particularly important for discussing Fourier systems. We see that "Fourier analysis" is the process of starting with a wave and computing its constituents, including the type (sine or cosine) of wavelets, their amplitudes (coefficients), and their frequencies. In effect, Fourier analysis begins with the whole—a wave—and determines its parts—a series of weighted wavelets.

67

Of course the motivation here is the same as in Zernike systems. We seek to deduce the constituent aberrations in the optics of an eye. However, Fourier analysis provides a list of weighted wavelets in a wavefront (treated as a wave) rather than a list of weighted polynomials in a wavefront (treated as a shape). And yes, waves do have shapes, but we will see that the mathematics and methodology are quite different.

219. We recall that—upon successful analysis—Zernike polynomials are identified and listed according to their indices, as in the graph in paragraph 192. *A corresponding graph for a Fourier system*—upon analysis—*identifies and lists wavelets according to their frequencies.* Hence we say that the latter graph is in a frequency domain and that it shows a "frequency spectrum." (See paragraph 207.) Both Zernike polynomials and Fourier wavelets are quantified by coefficients, but a point to be emphasized later is that Fourier frequencies are handled differently than Zernike indices in order to be clinically applicable.

Though this notion is also of interest to students of the "beauty" in mathematics, we rely on the fact that Fourier analysis elegantly converts information in the space domain into information in the frequency domain. In particular, the space domain reveals wavefronts as waves. The frequency domain reveals constituent wavelets which are identified by their frequencies (and quantified by their coefficients). As noted, the frequency-domain representation can be made clinically utile, even though the various constituent frequencies correspond only indirectly to the various optical aberrations of the eye in question.

220. "Fourier synthesis" is the opposite process which starts with the constituent wavelets and yields a weighted sum representing the wave. In effect, Fourier synthesis sums the parts to assemble the whole. This process is easy to appreciate in terms of music: a complex musical sound can be synthesized by playing together several pure tones, each with some particular pitch (frequency) and loudness (amplitude).

221. We may also learn that Fourier analysis is a form of "harmonic analysis." This is true since sound waves lend themselves to Fourier analysis. We will say more about the connection to music later, but as will be apparent, Zernike analysis is quite different in this regard.

222. In a Fourier system, a *Fourier transform* (one of several kinds, and this term is a noun) can be used to facilitate finding the constituent wavelets and coefficients. Such a transform is the mathematical process or algorithm by which a Fourier series is obtained—in essence, *it performs Fourier analysis*—though sometimes the term is used for the result of that process. A Fourier transform is actually an integral equation in which the sines and cosines are expressed as exponents. This equation treats a wavefront as a wave, and it involves some means of finding best-fitting wavelets. With proper effort, it can also be digitalized.

We will use Fourier transforms later. We will look at their newer versions ("discreet" and "fast") and we will see how to use them, but for now suffice it that Fourier transforms are computer-compatible "tools" for analyzing waves into wavelets; that is to say, Fourier transforms are really only methods of Fourier analysis. We can add that such transforms facilitate the re-expression (the mathematical transformation without change in value) of a function from a time-domain or a space-domain representation to a representation in a frequency-domain, as explained above.

223. An *inverse Fourier transform* does the opposite. In Fourier systems, an inverse Fourier transform can recreate the wavefront out of constituent wavelets and coefficients. I.e., an inverse Fourier transform does efficient synthesis, and it obviously "runs backwards."

FOURIER SYSTEM EQUATIONS and the MASTER EQUATION

We turn to Fourier system equations. Admittedly, what follows again is mainly mathematical (algebraic and trigonometric), but that is "the nature of this beast." One consolation is that this is a prime example of beneficently applied mathematics.

224. The general Fourier "master equation" is as follows, which in effect reiterates the statement that "any wave can be reconstructed from a weighted sum of sinusoidal wavelets with different frequencies."

$$F(x) = a_o + \sum_{n=1}^{\infty} \left\{ a_n \cos(nx) + b_n \sin(nx) \right\}$$

Again let us dissect this for our purposes and mention certain nuances.

225. The term $F(x)$, in short, *represents the wave*. Here it is a function of x, which means it varies depending on the value of x. In general, x symbolizes location or distance, and we will see this in a graph. (See also paragraph 207 about domains.)

The wave can also be set up to be a function of time, and it is then expressed as $F(t)$. In other words if we think of frequency as how fast a wave repeats in some space, we use $F(x)$; if we think of how fast the wave repeats in a time interval, we use $F(t)$. The wave is said to be "periodic," and the period is the time (or space) for one oscillation.

Either way, $F(x)$ and $F(t)$ *can represent wavefronts in the Fourier system as wave functions*. The former representation is equivalent to the "wavefront aberration function" in the Zernike system, $W(\rho, \theta)$ or $W(x,y)$, as in paragraph 39. The space-domain form of the Fourier function, $F(x)$, is more important for us, because we generally do not consider a wavefront in a time domain. See Note 7 on page 89.

In terms of an *x-y* system of coordinates in a graph, $F(x)$ is simply the value on the *y* axis that corresponds to a value of x along the *x* axis. (See the review on *x-y* coordinates in paragraph 205.) Of course we can start anywhere along *x* but by tradition we start at the point where $y = 0$. Likewise we can start anywhere along *y*, and that point is the *y* "intercept." The wave in a graph can be the sum of several smaller waves along the same horizontal axis; see paragraph 254. Indeed the gist of the mathematical breakthrough in Fourier's mathematics is how waves can be combined to create new waves, and we will see examples of how this is done and how it can be used.

226. The next part of the above equation is a_0. Mathematically, it is the average (mean) value of $F(x)$ or $F(t)$ over one cycle, which portends that it has a similar (but not identical) role to the zero mean of polynomials in Zernike systems, as in paragraph 106. More noticeably in a graph, a_0 controls the up-down position of the wave relative to the (horizontal) x axis; if a_0 is zero, the wave is centered on the x axis, and a_0 may be omitted from the equation. For example, since the x axis in the diagram in paragraph 235 is set at zero (where $y = 0$), then $a_0 = 0$ in the corresponding Fourier equation. In short, a_0 can be the y intercept. When the up-down position matters, two conventions exist for specifying this, either by including a_0 or by including $\dfrac{a_0}{2}$ in the equation; the choice is an issue of preference, and we should not be confused when we see Fourier equations written either way. (In the second convention, a_0 is twice the mean.) Thus in the diagram in paragraph 75, where the x axis represents 2 meters, a_0 (or $\dfrac{a_0}{2}$) would not be zero in the corresponding Fourier equation, in which case the mean value of the coefficients is not zero.

227. The $\displaystyle\sum_{n=1}^{\infty}$ means addition or summation. The infinity sign indicates that, at least in theory, an endless number of terms can be added together. Starting with 1, the n shows the numbering of these terms. However, a more pertinent interpretation of n is this. In Fourier synthesis we add more and more terms—meaning more and more wavelets—in order to arrive at a sufficiently complete rendition of the wave. In effect *we repeatedly solve the above equation for $F(x)$, adding more detail each time.* The repetitions are called *"iterations,"* and the n identifies the iteration (first, second, etc.) Ideally, the highest n is reached when further iterations add only inconsequential details.

228. This is a key concept in the Fourier system worth emphasizing: *Our total picture of the wavefront is built out of many wavelets.* We will see that in general—because of the declining coefficients associated with each successive wavelet—each iteration adds a smaller and smaller detail to that picture, as the entire weighted sum "converges" on the desired endpoint.

Think of paying off $99.99 first with twenties, then adding a ten-dollar bill, then adding a five, then adding ones, then adding quarters, dimes, etc., as the payments "converge" on $99.99. To extend this analogy, the value of each bill or coin is a "frequency," and each addition of another piece of money is an iteration. Moreover, each subsequent denomination is smaller, which means that it fits more times into $99.99; i.e., it has a "higher frequency." The number of each denomination needed—for example 4 twenties—roughly represents the "coefficient" or "amplitude" of that "frequency." (We used this analogy in paragraph 143. Of course the analogy does not illustrate infinite detail, but we usually stop at approximately 60 iterations; we will return to this point.)

229. Despite the dissimilarities, the above methodology is reminiscent of a Zernike system. Each additional Zernike polynomial, weighted by a coefficient, adds more detail to a sum until an adequate endpoint is reached for the accurate representation of the overall refractive status. The approximate Fourier counterparts of Zernike "orders" are iterations. That is to say, high-order Zernike aberrations in general require many Fourier iterations in order to converge on the sought-after endpoint, though orders are not exactly the same as iterations. We will return to this difference because it has practical significance.

230. This brings us to the all-important coefficients, the a's and b's in the above master equation. (Technically, a_0 is also a coefficient, but we can sidestep this issue.) *The Fourier coefficients tell us how strong or "weighty" a contribution each wavelet makes to the wave, and Fourier coefficients are equivalent to Zernike coefficients, usually labeled as C's, which also tell us how much of each aberration afflicts the eye.* In this sense, determining the a's and b's in Fourier analysis is the key step—and also the most difficult. (Moreover, Fourier uses these two kinds of coefficients.)

The a's customarily modify the cosine wavelets, and the b's the sine wavelets. In any one equation, each a_n and b_n is unique, and as mentioned, they generally tend to decrease in each successive iteration. Coefficients can be computed, though this requires some calculus. (See Note 8 on page 89.)

231. As for the "sin" and "cos" in the above basic equation, of course they refer to how the wavelets are generated trigonometrically. The quantities of which we find the sine or cosine, the "(nx)'s" in the above equation, are products of n and other numbers which we will get to shortly.

232. Sine and cosine waves are very basic, found in countless physical and mathematical processes (as in paragraph 79 for the Zernike system). It is possible to write the above equation as just a sine equation or just a cosine equation by incorporating the phase difference between sines and cosines. Moreover, certain waves can be built from just sine wavelets or just cosine wavelets.

233. However, both are needed if a phase difference between wavelets needs to be specified, i.e., if a left-to-right shift is significant before the wavelet is added to the sum. This shift is achieved by a combination of a sine wavelet and a cosine wavelet in appropriate proportions. Here we recall (paragraphs 180 - 182) that Zernike systems specify any axis of astigmatism, or of any other meridional aberration such as tilt, coma, etc., through a combination of two similar polynomials which differ by their orientation in space. We will return to this point for Fourier systems in a more meaningful setting.

234. It also helps to know that by the application of some trigonometry these sines and cosines can be expressed as exponents. Though the above general equation captures the essence of Fourier's mathematics, the actual analysis of waves into wavelets is usually done by using some form of Fourier transform, which is an equation built of exponents. We should therefore not be astonished to see exponential equations in the literature on Fourier transforms. (Indeed exponential equations are often easier to manage than sin/cosine equations, even if the former are less intuitive and generally less familiar.)

235. Now we turn to the last element of each cos and sin term, the frequency *nx*, which as we pointed out is how wavelets are identified. The coefficients give the weight of each wavelet, while the frequencies identify each wavelet. Frequency is the most intricate item, in part because frequency can be expressed in several ways. Here we need the help of a graph of a typical wavelet, as in the diagram; it is a sine wave, though of course a cosine wave would be just as legitimate.

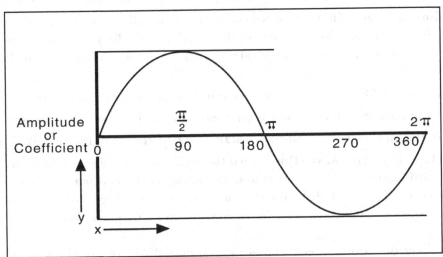

A wavelet which is a sine wave. The *x* axis is marked in degrees and radians. One complete cycle covers 360 degrees, which is 2π radians. The *y* axis is the amplitude, or in our context, the coefficient. Since this wave consists of one complete cycle, its frequency is one (1).

236. The diagram shows a wavelet completing one cycle within the given "space," though wavelets (and waves in general) can complete one or more cycles within that "space." In order to make wavelets comparable, we normalize them so that they fit into that "space." The wavelets will then fill the entire allotted length of the *x* axis. The "space" along the *x* axis is equivalent to one circumference of a circle; we can think of it as one cycle or one go-around. However, one cycle can also be a period of time. (Hence the quotes around "space.") In any case, *the number of complete wavelets that can fit into such a circle is the frequency.* This is the same idea as the meridional or azimuthal frequency in Zernike's system. Meanwhile, of course, wavelets with greater coefficients will be proportionally taller along the *y* axis in a graph of this kind.

Incidentally, normalization is different in the Fourier system than in the Zernike system, in part because of the uniform structure of wavelets compared to the varying structure of Zernike polynomials. Fourier normalization is not a major concern in our setting.

237.   Here is where cross-comparisons become problematic, and we brought up this issue in paragraph 225. If an author expresses frequency in terms of space, we may see an x, (and usually an $F(x)$, as in our equation above and the diagram) or we may see the "wave number" k, which is 2π per wave length, or other labels for distance. Furthermore we may encounter $\omega_0 t$ or other labels. The symbol ω_0 indicates angular frequency, which is a measure of the speed at which the wave cycles (degrees or radian per second), so that $\omega_0 t$ actually is also a distance. (Think of "speed times time equals distance.") The subscript $_0$ refers to the initial frequency; i.e., the frequency of the wavelet in the first iteration. The reason we present this detail is that it points to a logical way with which to explain the following concept.

238.   The n, as in "$n\,\omega_0\,t$," is the iteration number, which means that the *wavelet's frequency increases at each iteration*. In other words with each successive iteration, the wavelet cycles more times in the same distance, and that distance is $\omega_0 t$ (or 2π in the graph). If the initial frequency (that of the first wavelet) is f, then the frequency of the second wavelet is $2f$, and that of the third wavelet is $3f$, etc. At times, depending on the mathematical circumstances, only odd or even n's are included, but they are integers (no fractions). We note that by introducing frequencies, the stage is set for conversion into a frequency domain.

239.   Recalling the notion of convergence (paragraph 228), we can think of iterations as successive tries to converge on $F(x)$ as completely as possible. With each iteration, the system "tries" a *more compact wavelet*, one with more cycles per space. Meanwhile, *with each iteration, the coefficient usually shrinks*. As will be illustrated, the coefficient may be the reciprocal of the iteration number, so that if the initial coefficient (for the first wavelet) was 1, in the coefficient for the next wavelet may be $\frac{1}{2}$. Then the coefficient of the next wavelet it may be $\frac{1}{3}$, etc. ("May be" because in many cases not every wavelet is evaluated, and the coefficients need not always be reciprocals of the frequencies.)

WAVES, WAVEFRONTS and FOURIER EXPANSIONS

240. Now a more complete paradigm emerges. Like we "analyzed" $99.99 with smaller and smaller denominations, *we analyze the wave—which, lest we forget, describes the wavefront—by adding incrementally faster but incrementally smaller wavelets.* By "faster" we mean higher frequency.

241. But here another concept needs to be introduced, one which we applied in the Zernike system (in paragraph 155) and which we will expand upon later: Using the $99.99 analogy, after the first iteration with four twenties we have paid $80.00. Had we stopped there, we would have a "*residual*" of $19.99. After the next iteration with a ten-dollar bill, the residual is only $9.99, and the process is repeated—"iterated"—with incrementally smaller denominations. Just a few iterations suffice to shrink the residuals to nothing, at which time we reach—we have converged on—our goal. We have found the "best-fitting" denominations.

242. When wavelets are added together, the addition is "algebraic" in the sense that a negative term can be "added" in. Think of it this way: our debt was $99.99, we "converged" only to $99.05, so the residual is $0.04. An expeditious final step is to pay with a nickel and then take back (subtract) a cent. We can also say that we overestimated our debt and need to retract our payment somewhat. Upon adding 5 cents, a *negative* residual has been temporarily incurred. In the Fourier system this circumstance arises when a wavelet is added that is too large; "adding" the next smaller wavelet as a negative amount achieves the compensation. This is a reason we see Fourier equations (and Zernike equations; see paragraphs 88 to 91) with negative terms.

243. Now let us think again of a large debt, because then a problem will be encountered. How do we know where to start? With thousand-dollar bills or with hundreds? Moreover, are nickels and pennies even needed? I.e., which denominations are best for the process? In terms of best wavelets, with which frequencies should the wave be sampled? The reason for this part of the analogy is this. A practical issue in the Fourier system is that an algorithm "samples" the wave by use of sine and/or cosine wavelets to analyze the wave (with a computer program).

244. Worded more formally, a general problem in the analysis of waves is that the sampling must be done at a high enough frequency so that loss of detail is minimized. In this case, at what sampling frequency does the system offer good *fidelity* so that it can reconstruct a wavefront which faithfully represents the true refractive status? It turns out that the frequency of sampling should be at least twice the maximum frequency of the wave being sampled, while the latter can be pre-estimated. (In clinical practice, there is an expected range in frequency, because the human wavefront very rarely has steep gradients or slopes.)

This rule is "Nyquist's sampling theorem," and as it implies, higher sampling frequency allows better fidelity, which in theory translates into better resolution of the details in a wavefront. It so happens that Fourier's system can use a sampling frequency beyond the Nyquist frequency, which should allow very good fidelity. In the money analogy, a Fourier system can select the appropriate denominations so that the final sum can be accurately and efficiently deduced. Inadequate sampling introduces an error called "aliasing" (though the term has other technological meanings). Sampling with wavelets of excessive frequency wastes the system's resources and time.

245. This is not a major issue in Zernike's system, in part because Zernike polynomials are pre-structured with the shape of the wavefront in mind. Nevertheless a kind of sampling is involved, as the Zernike system also analyzes an overall aberration by "trying out" many simpler aberrations. However, it uses polynomials which specifically describe either clinically familiar aberrations (e.g., "astigmatism") or more exotic optical aberrations. Fourier polynomials only describe wavelets.

◆

246. We continue this section by "expanding" the basic Fourier equation to show the historically most famous Fourier series. In this case a step-like "wave," which has straight lines and sharp corners, is constructed by the summation of obviously curved sine or cosine wavelets. The "expanded" equation, to be compared with the master equation (paragraph 224), shows each term separately, as follows.

$$F(t) = \sin(\omega_0 t) + \frac{1}{3}\sin(3\,\omega_0 t) + \frac{1}{5}\sin(5\,\omega_0 t) + \frac{1}{7}\sin(7\,\omega_0 t)\ldots\ .$$

We use "$\omega_0 t$" here and show four terms, i.e., four iterations.[11] The coefficient of the first term, as well as its n, are understood to be 1. Here all n's and coefficients are odd, to be explained later.

247. The point is that each successive iteration shows a smaller coefficient ($\frac{1}{3}$, $\frac{1}{5}$, $\frac{1}{7}$ ...) and a larger frequency (e.g., 3, 5, 7...), in agreement with the principle that the series "converges" on the wave. Here that wave is shown as a function of time ($F(t)$). Nonetheless, *all terms are identical* except for two numbers; no matter how many iterations are involved, each term is structured as "$b_n \sin(n\omega_0 t)$," and if cosine terms were called for, as "$a_n \cos(n\omega_0 t)$." In contrast, as explained earlier, one of the problems with Zernike polynomials is that they tend to become more complex for higher orders.

248. In this instance the first wavelet of course is a simple sine wave, as in diagram 235, and as incredible as it seems, after enough iterations the wave looks like this (diagram on next page):

---

[11] Since each term is also a function that contributes to the sum, each can be called a "basis function." This terminology stems from vector algebra, which can be used on Fourier series. The analogous term applies to the Zernike system.

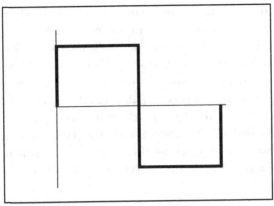

A square "wave" constructed from many
sinusoidal wavelets. Note straight lines and
right-angled "square" corners.

249. The intermediate steps, not essential for us, would consume much space and require additional explanations as well as diagrams. These can be found in almost all sources on Fourier mathematics, e.g., http://mathworld.wolfram.com/FourierSeriesSquareWave.html. Still, we note that waves with *straight lines* can be built from sinusoidal wavelets, which implies that the Fourier system can deal with straight lines. Later we will see how this point is clinically pertinent.

250. Incidentally, as clever as Fourier was, some of his reputable mathematical colleagues at first derided this idea. How can squared waves be produced out of obviously curved waves? That is to say, by analogy, how can a square hole be made out of round holes? But once we picture it, the idea is remarkably simple: drill many smaller and smaller round holes. The relevance for us is two-fold. First, any wavefront can be made from—and consists of—enough smaller and smaller sinusoidal wavelets. Second, rectilinear shapes are possible. Consider the following diagram, which indeed in a graphic sense symbolizes the above equation.

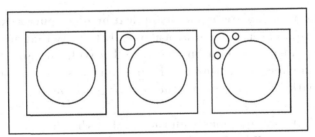

A square hole is made from smaller and smaller
round holes. With enough such holes any shape,
even a square, can be easily produced.

251. Before leaving this case, let us also mention two miscellaneous technical details. For one, all terms—all Fourier polynomials (like all Zernike polynomials)—are "orthogonal," which means they are mathematically independent. This feature is essential to the formation of weighted sums, and it also plays the same role in best-curve fitting.

252. In addition, a Fourier expansion may contain consecutively numbered terms, as in the preceding example, or it may only consist of just even-numbered or odd-numbered terms (as some amplitudes can be zero). This peculiarity follows rules which are rarely vital in our context, but some details are helpful in comparing Fourier equations and waves. If a wavelet is symmetric with respect to the y axis, its coefficient is even-numbered and it is a cosine function. This is mirror-image symmetry. If the wavelet's *inflection* is symmetric about the y axis, e.g., if the right upper quadrant is like the left lower quadrant flipped over, it is a sine function with an odd coefficient. This is inflection symmetry; the diagram below shows the two kinds of symmetry. Some wavelets are neither exclusively even nor odd, but they may be decomposed into a sum of both. Furthermore, terms can be negative or positive, as mentioned.

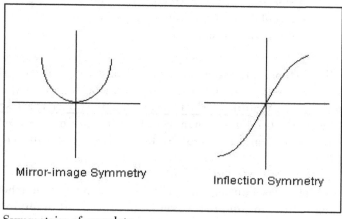

Mirror-image Symmetry · Inflection Symmetry

Symmetries of wavelets.

✦

253. We can now focus on a more practical application of a Fourier expansion, but one that in principle is like the square wave case shown above. Let us say that our equipment, including a H-S device, has provided raw data on the overall wavefront, and then some integrated computerized device in effect has performed Fourier analysis on this data so that we can see what we are dealing with. The diagram on the next page will help.

254. We assume that our equipment informs us that the shape of a particular wavefront consists of the weighted sum only of three wavelets. (In reality this is unlikely. We will use a broader clinical example later after covering other technicalities.) For clarity, the applicable expanded equation is spread out as follows.

$$\sin(\omega_0 t) \;+\; \frac{1}{2}\sin(2\omega_0 t) \;+\; \frac{1}{3}\sin(3\omega_0 t) \;=\; F(t)$$

which in words—and in the following diagram—is equivalent to

'first iteration + second iteration + third iteration = total wave.'

255.   The above equation is the same type we saw in paragraph 246, though the graphic result is quite different; it certainly does not have straight lines or corners. We note that the three wavelets are sine waves, each of lesser amplitude and greater frequency. Each represents additional detail on the refractive status. When all three waves are added together, the result is the 'total wave,' representing the overall refractive error in the diagram. This total wave is akin to the kind of wave we might find—at least in theory—when analyzing raw data from our aberrometry.

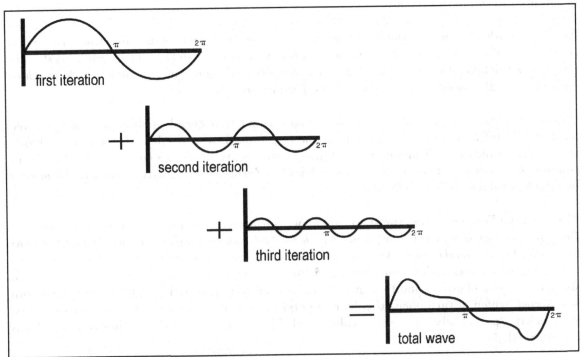

A Fourier expansion and synthesis of a 'total wave' from three wavelets according to the equation above. Each wavelet is an iteration.

256.   This brings us to a subtle but practically significant difference between Zernike orders and Fourier iterations; we touched on this point in paragraphs 144 and 229. Up to a limit, we can readily specify how many orders a Zernike system should include. In other words we can tell it where to stop. In so doing, we voluntarily exclude certain more complex refractive errors, since we bar their polynomials (as is clearer when polynomials are listed by the single-index method). This ability provides some clinical control over how much detail appears in the reconstruction of the wavefront.

In contrast, limiting the number of iterations in a Fourier system is not quite the same as limiting the orders in a Zernike system. Each subsequent Fourier polynomial does not correspond to a specific refractive error but only to additional resolution of the wavefront. This means that if our goal is to exclude negligible details about the wavefront (think of ignoring small change in a large debt), the Fourier system may be more precise.

78

DATA POINTS in FOURIER SYSTEMS

257. Let us now turn to data collection in a Fourier system. Data collection—data "acquisition" in some scientific circles but "aberrometry" in this case—is covered earlier in typical presentations, but to me it seems easier to know something about the math beforehand. Actually our commercially available aberrometry equipment has been quite similar in both systems—Zernike and Fourier—for several years, involving reflected retinal light, lenslets, a reference plane, video sensors, and a computerized algorithm. In fact, a H-S aberrometer can be adapted to run both systems.

258. In both systems the shape of the wavefront can be expressed as a function. However, there is a distinction according to how such a function is interpreted. The Zernike system in effect asks the following question. *Which polynomials—which refractive errors—can be weighted and added together so as to account for the wavefront aberration function?*

On the one hand, as a part of this scheme the most important Zernike polynomials are equated with named refractive errors; no separate naming procedure is needed. On the other hand, these polynomials are all predetermined and all different; some are simple and others very complicated. These and other conditions restrict the Zernike system with respect to the *method* by which the data are best collected.

259. In the Fourier system the shape of the wavefront is in the form of a wave function, and the Fourier system asks this question. *Which wavelets can be weighted and added together so as to account for the (total) wave?* On the one hand these wavelets are not immediately equated with refractive errors without another algorithm, but on the other hand they are all simple and similar. These and other conditions allow the Fourier system more latitude in *how the data can be collected*, which in turn opens the door to potentially better assessment of refractive errors. We can say "potentially," since the evolution of this field is rapid and the clinical implications are not settled.

260. This brings us to the details in the methods of data collection: *One major difference in the Fourier system is that more lenslets and therefore more spots—more "data points"—can be employed.* In general—and depending in part on pupil size—a Fourier system can gather data from 240 spots, vs. from about 40 in the Zernike system. This point is better made in reverse: *A principal limitation in the Zernike system compared with Fourier is significantly fewer usable data points.*

261. As we suggested earlier, an important corollary to this issue is that more sophisticated mathematical processes for deciphering the shape of the wavefront from the data can be applied in a Fourier system. We will come back to this point momentarily, but first we should review two main reasons for the difference in spot number (e.g., 240 vs. 40): First, in Fourier systems oval pupils do not reduce the number of useable data points. Second, data from two adjacent locations is not required for each determination of a local slope.

262. We already described the first of these reasons in paragraph 211, though it is less important. In short, the Zernike system excludes data points outside a perfect circle, such as those from an oval pupil, while the human pupil is rarely perfectly circular.

263. The second factor is more significant and more intricate. We recall (paragraph 36) that in a geometric sense a wavefront is a collection of many local slopes. In a H-S device, the acquisition of local slopes hinges on precise measurements of aberration-induced displacements of centroids, which are the points of maximum brightness of spots. These measurements take place in arrays of sensors (detector pixels), usually in a square pattern. Each array is a subaperture, and the difference in how much illumination two adjacent sensors receive quantifies the slope in this subaperture (paragraph 34). Given the small arena, this mechanism demands very precise technology, while the algorithm includes a form of mathematical integration across each subaperture.

264. One concern is that if the displacements are so large or the subapertures so small that a spot from one lenslet illuminates another's subaperture, the algorithm may report spurious results. In addition, the spots cannot be too spread out, lest they straddle too many sensors. Clearly the requirement for an acceptable size of subapertures limits the number of spots and subapertures, especially when severe aberrations can give rise to large displacements. Another issue is that some peripheral subapertures may be cleaved by the edge of the array of subapertures, so that these spots may not contribute useable data.

265. The Fourier system, in contrast, is compatible with reconstruction of the wavefront from wave-like displacements and from wave-like variations in the intensity of spots. For the calculation of slopes, the following principle can therefore be used: a flat wavefront allows a lattice-like pattern of about 240 evenly spaced and equally weighted centroids to be superimposed on the reference plane. This pattern is readily compatible with an ordinary two-dimensional Cartesian system of coordinates. When aberrations are present in an eye, *the shape of the wavefront can be gleaned—reconstructed—from distortions in the overall pattern rather than from individual locations.* Roughly speaking, each spot alone can be evaluated against whole two-dimensional Cartesian lattice, without data from an adjoining sensor.

We can think of this concept in terms of the diagram above paragraph 36, where we considered an arrangement with only 16 lenslets and 16 spots. If this were a Fourier system, all 16 spots could act in one large subaperture. Moreover, additional spots and detector pixels could be fitted into the area of the reference plane, while their alignment with the lenslets becomes less critical. (See Note 9 on page 89.) We can also say that Zernike's approach to wavefront reconstruction relies on local slopes whereas Fourier's approach, by its mathematical nature, uses global waves.

266. In mathematical terms, integration in Fourier analysis is carried out over the entire population of spots, not just individually, and the result allows direct construction of the wavefront. (See next diagram, and see equations 1 vs. 15 in Zon et al.) This pattern-distortion approach also suggests another quite different method of data collection called "curvature sensing," but we will take this up later so as not to interrupt the flow to the next topic, demodulation.

FOURIER DEMODULATION

267. The pattern-distortion approach is an application of *two-dimensional Fourier demodulation*. A non-medical example of demodulation is radio reception. A radio signal consists of a "carrier wave" which, in the absence of meaningful sound, is regular—equally spaced—in amplitude or in frequency (hence AM/FM). When sound is transmitted, a small "signal wave" is superimposed on the carrier wave. The receiver produces sound by extracting the irregular signal wave from the otherwise regular carrier wave; this process is demodulation, and it is "a natural" for Fourier analysis.

268. In our context, *demodulation accomplishes the extraction of two-dimensional irregularities—caused of course by optical aberrations—in the otherwise regular lattice-like pattern of spots on a reference plane.* In this setting the reference plane is the "Fourier plane," which is merely a focal plane of the eye. The irregularities or distortions or modulations on this plane are treated as a wave, though this would not work if the irregularities were extreme. (Even with some pupil centroid misalignment, the distortions are practically unchanged, which may make the system somewhat more robust.) We note how the intensity of the spots shows the distortion, as in this example. (See Note 10 on page 90.) We also see that a Cartesian system of coordinates, rather than a spherical polar system, works well in this arrangement, even though far more than 40 spots are considered.

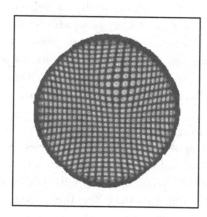

Distortion of spots on a reference plane from an eye with aberrations (actual photograph). The distorted pattern clearly is wave-like, even in this two-dimensional view. Without distortions, the pattern would be a regular Cartesian grid.

269. The sensitivity of this kind of system to distortions in the pattern means that the emmetropic pattern—with no aberrations at all—ideally should consist of a perfectly regular pattern made up of identical centroids. As we will mention again when listing the disadvantages of Fourier systems, such perfection is technically difficult to maintain.

270. Once all the raw data have been collected and demodulated so that the shape of the wavefront has been reconstructed into a wave, this wave can be Fourier-analyzed with respect to its constituent wavelets. The algorithm for extracting the identity and magnitude of these wavelets from the wavefront may go as follows (though again alternatives exist).

1. Try a reasonable wave—a wavelet, really—as the first iteration; the frequency of this "test wave" can exceed the Nyquist frequency (since maximum frequency is known).
2. Calculate the residual. In effect, "see how close we came" with the test wave.
3. Treat the residual as new data—after all, the residual itself is a wave—and re-test with a wavelet of higher frequency.
4. Repeat the process—continue iterations—until the residual is expected to be negligible, which may be assumed to be the case after about 60 iterations.
5. Stop sooner if residuals become negligible sooner. (The capacity of the system to stop automatically means that pre-setting by the operator may not be necessary.)
6. Gather successful wavelets (with amplitudes); these are the constituents of the wavefront.

271. This process invites a question: how does the system find the best-fitting wavelets? The answer in most programs—but not in all—consists of some form of searching for best fits. In principle, the procedure (paragraph 155) can be similar to the one in Zernike systems, but of course a Fourier system deals with wavelets. Since a wavelet is a curve, the exercise amounts to "best-curve fitting," though the general principle can be illustrated on a "straight curve," i.e., a straight line, and then extrapolated to accommodate curves. Fourier transforms aid the process, but no matter how it is achieved, *the outcome should be a set of constituent sinusoidal wavelets which "best-fit" the wave.* Of course clinical use of this set requires more work, to which we will return.

272. Here again is where orthogonality of wavelets (their mathematical independence) is crucial, because this feature allows each wavelet to be best fit no matter how many others are involved. This means that the amplitude—and hence the coefficient—can accurately and independently reflect the amount of each aberration that is involved.

◆

273. Let us briefly elaborate on the connection between musicology and Fourier math—mentioned in paragraphs 220 and 221—as this connection is informative. A complex musical note can be synthesized from pure-tone sine wavelets, and it can be analyzed into its constituent pure-tone sine wavelets. Both processes obey Fourier synthesis and analysis.

When one piano key is struck—say, middle C—the instrument emits a complex note which consists of a wave with a frequency of (usually) 256 cycles per second, as well as a series of wavelets—overtones—each less loud (lower amplitude) but higher in pitch (greater frequency). The wave is called the "fundamental" or the "first harmonic," and it corresponds to the "test wave" in the above algorithm. The subsequent wavelets correspond to the second, third, fourth, etc., harmonics. The frequency of each is a multiple of the frequency of the first, while the amplitude declines by the same proportion. For instance, a wavelet, representing the fifth harmonic, with a frequency which is 5 times greater than that of the fundamental, will have 1/5th the amplitude, etc.

This mechanism (which is the heart of music theory, harmony, dissonance, and tonality) is exactly what we rely on when we analyze wavefronts in a Fourier system. In this sense, Fourier analysis describes mathematically how a musicologist listening to an entire orchestra can tell who has played what at which pitch and loudness. As an alternative model, our equipment "listens" to the "orchestra" of the optics of the eye and reports the loudness and pitch of each constituent tone.

CURVATURE SENSING

274.   Before leaving the topic of data collection, let us discuss another way to reconstruct the wavefront based on relative intensities; we touched on this already in paragraph 266. It is an example of how a Fourier system is more amenable than a Zernike system to a variety of technical approaches which hold promise for improved performance.

The traditional H-S device senses local slopes for reconstructing the shape of the wavefront in a time-tested and logical manner, one which arose in the design of astronomic telescopes. The pertinent fact is that the detection of slopes occurs on a reference plane which is perpendicular to the optical axis. I.e., the intensities of spots are compared at various locations on one frontal plane. However, if rays of light pass through *two* reference planes along the optical axis, the intensity may be different at each plane. *This difference is proportional to—and therefore is also a measure of—the local curvature.*

275.   In more detail, two blurred images are formed, one just anterior to the focal plane (the pre-focal or intra-focal image) and the other just posterior (post-focal or extra-focal). In the absence of aberrations, the two images are practically equal in intensity. Now let us imagine that the rays for these images arise from a localized corneal lesion; think of a bump on the wavefront. In that case one of the two images will be brighter than the other. For instance, a convexity makes the post-focal image brighter, and the amount of difference in intensity indicates how much convexity exists at this point. The analysis proceeds point-by-point. This arrangement is called the Beckers-Roddier curvature sensor, and the basic distinction between it and H-S is simple: H-S measures side-to-side displacements; Beckers-Roddier measures front-to-back displacements. See diagram which follows.

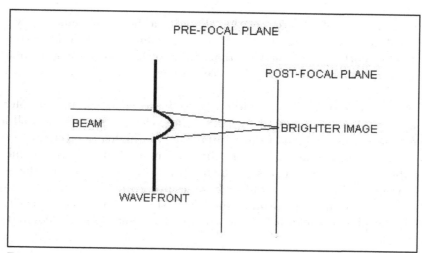

Diagrammatic side view of a Beckers-Roddier curvature sensor. A beam (from left) has an aberration which causes a convexity on the wavefront. The image of the spot is brighter on the post-focal plane than on the pre-focal plane.

276. A key equation here defines the "Laplacian operator," [12] so the result is the "Laplacian curvature," and the process is called *"curvature sensing,"* as distinguished from H-S "gradient sensing." This distinction however is not absolute; the Laplacian equation quantifies the changes in a gradient, so that in a sense both methods deal in gradients. Moreover, the slopes of the wavefront at the edge of the pupil (where the Laplacian operator does not apply) are derived during curvature sensing. Still, *curvature sensing provides enough information to reconstruct the wavefront.*

Using standard labels, I is the intensity, energy, or brightness; x and y are two dimensions; ∂ means partial differential; and ∇ stands for the gradient. To define his operator in Cartesian coordinates, Laplace wrote $\nabla^2 I = \frac{\partial^2 I}{\partial x^2} + \frac{\partial^2 I}{\partial y^2}$ which in effect gives the "slope of the slope" of intensity (a second partial differential).

277. The critical observation is that the difference in intensity is related to the Laplacian operator. (To be precise, it is proportional to the Laplacian of the "phase" of the wavefront, since light travels in phases, like soldiers marching in step, but we need not detour for this point.) If the difference in intensity is ΔI, and the Laplacian operator is $\nabla^2 I$, then (approximately) $\Delta I / I = \nabla^2 I$, ignoring an (ordinary derivative) term for the pupil edge. It turns out that *the wavefront can be Fourier-synthesized from* $\nabla^2 I$. (A Laplacian curvature is also a wave.) The wavelets and their coefficient are then within easy reach with the aid of a Fourier transform.

The main advantage of this method is a comparative immunity to technical artifacts. Also, some of the components in a H-S device can be used in curvature sensing. For more information, several web sites help; see Note 11 on page 90. However, to date most refractive surgery systems still rely on the traditional H-S/gradient approach. A third approach, shear interferometry, is beyond our scope here.

✦

278. Returning to the main line of Fourier systems, let us assume that the appropriate algorithm has extracted those frequencies which exist in the reconstructed wave, so that the wavefront for this eye is a known set of constituent sinusoidal frequencies; we then have a Fourier series of wavelets. Let us further assume that an algorithm has determined an amplitude (a coefficient) and a phase (incidental here) for each constituent wavelet. As we know, each frequency identifies a wavelet, while the amplitude quantifies the wavelet. Moreover, we know the relationship between successive iterations and (declining) amplitudes. From here, the clinical parallel is straightforward: the total refractive error is a sum of constituent errors, each quantified by a coefficient.

---

[12] Operators are complicated mathematical commands. A simple operator is "+."

279.   Earlier (paragraphs 254-255) we saw the mathematics of a hypothetical wave made of three sine wavelets. Let us examine two additional cases which are more instructive for the clinical setting. In the first case, we assume the eye has one refractive error, +3.00 hyperopia. Here the wavefront is represented by a wave which is a part of one unique sine wave. The system was normalized so that its amplitude is 2 (+1 above the x axis, -1 below the x axis; see paragraph 236 with the nearby diagram).

In a three-dimensional representation, the wavefront looks like a mound, while its two-dimensional representation in a graph (its profile) is half a sine curve; the frequency is ½ of 2π, which is just π. The "list" of best-fitting wavelets of course will turn out to consist of just one sine function with an amplitude of 2 and a frequency of π. An additional step—more on this shortly—can tell us that "$2 \sin \pi$" means "+3.00 hyperopia," so that we know that *100% of the refractive error in this eye, represented by 2 sin π , is +3.00 hyperopia*. Of course "$2 \sin \pi$" describes one wavelet.

280.   In the second case, the eye has two refractive errors, say, +2.00 hyperopia, and some lesser aberration, the identity of which does not matter. In a three-dimensional representation, the wavefront is *in part* a less-convex mound, so that its two-dimensional representation still includes half a sine curve. In other words the frequency is still ½ of 2π or just π , but the amplitude is less.

281.   However, the wavefront would embrace another deformation because of the presence of the second aberration, though this second deformity has a small amplitude and high frequency. The list of best-fitting wavelets will now turn out to contain *two* members: a sine function with an amplitude of 1.33 and a frequency of π , plus another sinusoidal function with amplitude 0.66 and a frequency of 2π. (We note that $1.33 + 0.66 \cong 2$, the normalized amplitude, so that the corresponding coefficients can be easily compared.) Now we know that *about two-thirds of the aberration is +2.00 hyperopia, and about one third is the other lesser aberration.*

Let us keep in mind that the two wavelets contribute to describe two shapes which are added together to form a new wave, that of the wavefront. The same concept applies in the Zernike system, as in paragraph 83, where shapes described by Zernike polynomials are added to each other.

282.   We note that Fourier wavelets (as in the diagram with paragraphs 254-255) are polynomials which conform to the pattern " $b_n \sin(n\varpi_0 t)$ " or " $a_n \cos(n\varpi_0 t)$." There is nothing distinctive about these, and in particular none of them suggests a specific optical/clinical entity such as "astigmatism," "defocus," or anything else that sounds like an ocular defect. As mentioned, another algorithm (Zernike-based) and another program are needed to attach appropriate clinical names of aberrations to the corresponding wavelets. After all, Zernike was an optical engineer, even if not an ophthalmologist, whereas Fourier was neither.

283.   Still, we are reminded that Fourier wavelet terms are analogous to Zernike polynomials; their sum is weighted by coefficients which quantify the existing aberrations, and the weighted sum, the "wave" or $F(x)$, is equivalent to the aberration function, $W(x,y)$ or $W(\rho,\theta)$.

A FOURIER TIME-LINE

284.   Let us assemble a more complete time-line—though it is one of many possible time-lines—for the main steps we have discussed:

1.   Raw data is obtained from a H-S device.
2.   This data is subjected to Fourier demodulation to extract distortions in the pattern.
3.   Distortions are converted to a wave which represents the wavefront.
4.   An initial sinusoidal wavelet which exceeds Nyquist frequency is best-fit to wave data.
5.   The residual is subjected to best-fitting with another higher-frequency wavelet.
6.   Steps 4 and 5 are repeated for 60 iterations, unless the residual vanishes earlier.
7.   The list of best-fit wavelets is assembled, representing the aberrations found in the eye.
8.   The coefficient of each wavelet quantifies these aberrations.
9.   Where possible, common optical names are assigned to these aberrations.
10.   Clinically significant data are converted to useful outputs, as in Zernike systems.
11.   Aberration data—in the form of an ablation profile—are sent to a surgical device.

This scheme, and most of the other steps, require a computer running Fourier-solving software; Fourier analysis of a wave "on paper" is very labor-intensive. However, a computer program in general can only accept digitalized numbers, which means that the wave must be sampled at some fixed frequency in order to provide these numbers. This is where the Nyquist frequency again is important. Another problem is that the immediate computerized output is in exponential form and must be converted in order to be in the more familiar trigonometric sine/cosine form.

285.   Many different *Fourier transform* programs (and their inverse; paragraphs 222 and 223) can help execute the above scheme. This is a separate intricate topic, but several additional terms regarding transforms appear in the eye literature, particularly "DFT" and "FFT."

A Fourier transform is easier to apply if it is modified into a DFT (discreet Fourier transform), which takes a "divide and conquer" approach to reduce the otherwise huge number of steps. The strategy converts the original integral equation into smaller and easier numerical-sum equations, though this process imposes some limitations. A further improvement is any of several FFT's (fast Fourier transforms), which trim the algorithm down further but impose additional restrictions. We emphasize that these transforms are equations which facilitate Fourier analysis.

286.   For those interested, in the following equation the first and second parts (left of ≡)

$$F(\omega)=\int_{-\infty}^{+\infty} f(t)e^{-i\omega t}dt \equiv \int_{-\infty}^{+\infty} f(t)[\cos(\omega t)-i\sin(\omega t)]dt$$

constitute the original Fourier transform. The term $F(\omega)$ here is a function of angular frequency, as are wavelets, while $f(t)$ is a function of time, as are waves. This means that this equation performs the analysis of a wave by identifying wavelets of various frequencies in a frequency domain. The process entails arduous integration, but the DFT and FFT formats are equations with Σ (for summation) wherein numbers are simply added, which lends itself well to digitalization and computerization. (We note the exponents.) The third part of the above equation (to the right of the $\equiv$ sign) shows that the Fourier transform satisfies the "master equation" in paragraph 224. Indeed this equation is easier to interpret in reverse; the sine/cosine master equation on the right is equivalent to an exponential Fourier transform in the middle, which is solved as a wave function on the left. In the entire process, the best-fitting wavelets are identified and quantified.

✦

287. Besides these programs, we should mention another development that is becoming part of future Fourier-based systems; this is an alternative mathematical way to reconstruct wavefronts. Shortcuts are available which use the second derivative of each sine and cosine function for computing the Fourier coefficients from the gradients (local slopes) of the wavefront. (See Note 12 on page 90.) In somewhat more detail, local wavefront gradients captured from H-S data are used to generate a "first combined gradient field" which is then subjected to Fourier analysis (mathematically, by obtaining the first partial derivative). The result, called a "first reconstructed wavefront," yields the "first revised gradient field." This field is again subjected to Fourier analysis (obtaining the second partial derivative), which provides a "second reconstructed wavefront." This procedure can be repeated (iterated) until a satisfactory endpoint is reached, which is a high-fidelity final wavefront. Generally 10 iterations suffice.

288. In this process, reliance on the least-square method is obviated, and the occasional loss of data is tolerable. (Some substandard data points can be ignored.) Nonetheless, this process does not display the results in familiar clinical terms, such as a refraction and words like sphere, cylinder, etc. An additional algorithm is still needed for this purpose, which we turn to next.

✦

289. We can go back to the point (paragraphs 279 and 282) that an addendum is needed for clinical-mathematical correlations in the Fourier system. We note again that the Fourier system does not provide a two-index scheme as does Zernike. In the latter system, a coefficient may be labeled as, say, C_2^{-2}, which is associated with the Zernike polynomial Z_2^{-2}. Since we know the meaning of each common index, this polynomial is unambiguously described. In other words, Zernike seeks amounts of fixed and identified polynomials that fit the shape of the wavefront.

Unfortunately we cannot simply look at a Fourier wavelet and deduce a descriptive identity; they all look alike. Fourier systems yield amplitudes of unfixed and unnamed wavelets that make up a wave, and they only provide a weighted expansion (list) of these wavelets. This list can be set into a graph as in paragraph 192, but instead of polynomials, the horizontal axis shows *the frequencies of the constituent wavelets*, which is a presentation in the frequency domain. Such a list is therefore a "frequency spectrum," which is mathematically elegant but by itself not clinically useful.

Hence we need the aforementioned addendum to convert the information into customary ophthalmic terms. For this purpose an extra series of Zernike-based steps is invoked, which finds and reports (by name) the clinically-identified Zernike polynomials that exist in that Fourier list.

DISADVANTAGES and ADVANTAGES of FOURIER SYSTEMS

290.   Ultimately, Fourier systems provide the same information as a Zernike system (paragraphs 190 to 198). However, as already hinted, the Fourier system has disadvantages. The main practical drawback may be too much detail. For example, the Fourier system can be sensitive enough to detect areas of tear film break-up. It may also sense corneal mucus or even floaters. In a worst-case scenario, the ablation profile may be "fooled" so that the laser is directed to respond to a nonexistent optical error. Of course simply by taking repeated measurements such transitory defects may be diluted away, and modern wavefront sensors are programmed to reject potentially invalid data, but a risk of untoward ablation still exists.

291.   Stated in reverse, the lesser sensitivity of a Zernike system at high orders may also make it less sensitive to technically introduced misinformation. That is to say, a "smoothing" effect may make a Zernike system more forgiving, so that very high resolution in wavefront analysis is not necessarily desirable. Therefore, in the clinical setting a little less fidelity may be preferable, in that the price for high fidelity is a receptiveness to small errors, to extraneous data, or to inferior data.

292.   While "noise" and other artifacts are also a problem in Zernike systems, they are exaggerated in more sensitive Fourier systems and may overwhelm useful data at high iterations. This is a particularly serious problem if the data points provided by a H-S sensor are of inconsistent quality. The focus of the lenslets—which is difficult to control—is especially critical, as blurred or unevenly placed centroids can easily be "confused" with clinically significant distortions. We recall (from paragraph 269 and the diagram just prior to that paragraph) that Fourier systems respond to the distortion in the pattern of spots, which implies that without aberrations all centroids ideally should be identical and regular.

Though the details are complex, we can generalize. A major technical limitation in typical Zernike systems is squeezing many subapertures into a reference plane while avoiding interference between adjacent spots. A major limitation in typical Fourier systems is ensuring a perfectly regular pattern of spots on a reference plane in emmetropia so that distortions are accurately detected.

293.   In addition we can easily command a Zernike system to stop at some desired order, which excludes more complex refractive errors but may also help exclude unwanted detail.

294.   Finally, a Fourier system in many ways is more complicated. For example, an additional algorithm is needed to generate a clinically worded output. (See paragraph 289.)

✦

295.   As we also already suggested, and as proponents of Fourier systems emphasize, these systems have advantages over Zernike systems. These advantages are easier to list numerically.

1.   Clearly, more detail and better fidelity—at least in principle—should allow better recognition and more effective remediation of defects. Indeed, it appears that a Fourier system which accepts 240 spots through a 7-mm pupil, even if that pupil is not wholly round, gives as much detail as 20 Zernike orders. (The extra spots are a major factor.)

2.   In theory—and we stress *in theory*—and as various technical problems are solved by better tracking, iris registration, etc., there is no limit to the fidelity and resolution possible in a Fourier system. In contrast, the smoothing effect in a Zernike system at high orders imposes such a limit, and anything beyond ten orders appears to offer no significant clinical advantage, or it provides data beset by prohibitive artifacts. In fact six or eight orders is the usual practical limit.

3.   A more subtle advantage resides in the fact that Fourier mathematics—but not Zernike's—allows the recognition of straight linear defects, such as corneal striae and cap amputations. (See paragraph 249.)

4.   In the clinical setting, these advantages appear to make a significant difference in eyes with complex aberrations, disease, and/or previously surgery. In other words, despite the risk of including unwanted detail, a Fourier system may be clinically superior for difficult cases.

5.   Evidence exists (see Chernyak, cited below) that PSF's based on Fourier synthesis are more similar to subjective descriptions of a point than those based on Zernike synthesis.

6.   Finally, with respect to mathematics alone, a Fourier system is not slowed or overloaded by very complex ("high-order," in Zernike terminology) aberrations and/or by measurements based on a large number of iterations. Reliance on Cartesian coordinates can reduce the number of iterations required for the evaluation of such aberrations, and as mentioned earlier, such coordinates work particularly well in Fourier systems.

296.   Nevertheless—as we pointed out at the start—as far as general clinical superiority is concerned, "the jury is still out," particularly for routine cases. We should also be aware that a Fourier system by itself offers no unique solutions to other problems in refractive surgery. For example, the technical dilemma remains that we determine the shape of the wavefront in the approximate plane of the pupil, yet our lasers ablate the anterior layers of the cornea. For another example, movements of the eye, including cyclotorsion and centroid shift, require attention in any case. Finally, no clinical application of either system remedies problems such as chromatic aberration, light-wave diffraction, or scattering of light.

✦

297.   For more mathematical information, a www search for "Fourier Analysis" or "Fourier Transform" will provide innumerable sites on various aspects of Fourier's work, but very few web sites are of direct relevance to ophthalmology. We should not be swayed by the well-publicized advantage which a Fourier system may offer in astronomic adaptive optics, where for example self-correcting telescopes are of great interest (ones which can quickly and automatically adjust for atmospheric turbulence). Though of course we hear less about these, advances in adaptive optics are of military interest, such as in the "star wars" program, but again few apply to ophthalmology. The Bibliography contains references on the Fourier system which do pertain to clinical practice and refractive surgery. The list is short, which in part is what prompted me to add to it.

NOTES

Including Helpful References

1. Much of this material was organized by the Optical Society of America. See a review by Thibos, Larry N., Indiana University. "Report from the VSIA Taskforce on Standards for the Reporting of the Optical Aberrations of the Eye." The extensive web site for this report is http://www.opt.indiana.edu/people/faculty/thibos/VSIA/VSIA-2000_taskforce/sld001.htm

2. Depending on the set-up, the front surface or face of a wavefront in the absence of aberrations can be convex (or similarly curved) rather than flat, because the eye is spherical. (See Figure 5 in Maeda, http://scien.stanford.edu/class/psych221/projects/03/pmaeda/index.html; full reference on page 94.) Think of a perimeter vs. a tangent screen. However, for simplicity we will consider the wavefront in the absence of aberrations to be flat. According to this convention, convexity is associated with defocus.

3. "Wavefront-guided" LASIK relies mainly on the shape of the wavefront. "Wavefront-optimized" LASIK relies more on standard refraction and past empirical data. Which of these is better for various kinds of refractive conditions is debatable and under study. For example see *EyeWorld Supplement*, "Wavefront Guided vs. Optimized." June 2006.

4. Orthogonal polynomials are at right angles to each other in a Cartesian system of coordinates and in vector form. The cross-product of orthogonal vectors is zero. Because they can be summed in this way, these polynomials are "linearly" independent.

5. An alternative definition of unit variance is via the equation (in spherical polar coordinates) $\frac{1}{N}\sum_{\rho,\theta}(W_{\rho,\theta} - Average)^2 = 1$ where N is the total number of errors.

6. Three examples appear in one article by Geipert, Nadja. "Fourier analysis - does better data equal better treatment?" in *ESCRS Eurotimes*, January 2006 issue (Volume II, Issue I, pages 1-3). The article contains clinical reports by D. Koch MD, J. Vukitch MD and M. Shabayek MD.

7. There is nothing peculiar about expressing a quantity in either a space domain or a time domain. We might say that something is "two blocks from here," or that it is "a five minute walk from here." We can generate a sine curve by measuring something at every centimeter (of space) or at every second (of time), but we customarily reconstruct wavefronts from slopes in space.

8. The coefficients a_0, a_n and b_n alone can be found by solving three integral equations based on a set of trigonometric-integral identities. For details and diagrams see *Wolfram* Math World, http://mathworld.wolfram.com/FourierSeries.html

9. See Zon N. et al. "Hartmann-Shack Analysis Errors." *Optics Express* Vol. 14, no. 2 (Jan. 2006): 635-643. Also see Canovas C. and Ribak E.N. "Comparison of Hartmann Analysis Methods" to be published in *Applied Optics*. These papers compare the centroid and Fourier demodulation methods.

90

10.   See extensive data in "Shack-Hartmann Wavefront Sensor for Laser Beam Analysis," http://shatura.laser.ru/WWW.LASER.RU/adopt/Science/sens/sensor.htm and Zavalova V. This web site is based on "Shack-Hartmann Wavefront Sensor for Beam Quality Measurements." *Optics for Industry and Medicine* (June 1997): 9-13.

11. See a PowerPoint presentation by So, Jonathan. "Adaptive Optics in Microscopy," optics.caltech.edu/ee131w05/reports/So2.ppt; also a brief review in University of Hawaii, http://www.ifa.hawaii.edu/ao/system/curv.html; and a more complete paper (still unpublished) in Optical Society of America, http://ol.osa.org/upcoming_pdf.cfm?id=67238.   Two crucial background papers (hard to find except as abstracts) are Roddier F. "Curvature Sensing: a new concept in adaptive optics." *Appl. Opt.* 27, 1988): 1223-1225; and the even more important Roddier F and Roddier C. "Wavefront Reconstruction Using Fourier Transforms." *Appl. Opt.* 30, (1991): 1327-1327. Also helpful is Barbero, S et al. "Wavefront Sensing and Reconstruction from Gradient and Laplacian Data Measured with a Hartmann-Shack Sensor." To be published by the Optical Society America, http://ol.osa.org/upcoming_pdf.cfm?id=67238.

12.   Personal communication, Douglas Koch MD and Dimitri Chernyak, Ph D. April 2006, and patent application (Chernyak et al.) in United States Patent Office, Washington DC, http://www.freshpatents.com/Iterative-fourier reconstruction for laser surgery and other optical applications dt20050120ptan20050012898.php.

BIBLIOGRAPHY

Where appropriate, annotations are provided to guide the reader in selecting additional sources. Otherwise, the format for the entries approximately follows the Chicago Manual of Style.[13]

REVIEW ARTICLES in WEB SITES on the ZERNIKE SYSTEM

For more information on Zernike, many excellent on-line reviews are readily available; here are examples, listed in approximate order of increasing complexity.

Pages 38-40 are a well-written very concise summary by Naeser, N. and Hjortdal, J, "Concepts of Regular Astigmatism in First Order Optics and Wave Front Analysis" which appears at http://www.saoa.co.za/publications/saoptom/2004/jan/journalvol63no1naeser.pdf

Another good concise summary by Tripoli, Nancy is in Opticon, "The Zernike Polynomials," at http://www.optikon.com/en/articles/keratron_023/media/TheAberrometers_2003_Tripoli%20(Zernike%20Polynomials).pdf

A visually appealing summary with clear slides by Thebos, Larry is in Indiana University, "Wavefront Data Reporting and Terminology," at their web site (which is linked to other articles) http://research.opt.indiana.edu/Library/VSIA/VSIA2001_tutorial/sld001.htm

Another good slide show (no author), "Basics of Zernike Expansion," which begins with the rudiments and includes diagrams copied in many other articles, is in the web site http://voi.opt.uh.edu/VOI/VSII%20-%20Slides%20of%20Lectures/Lecture%2014%20Zernike%20Expansion.pdf

Two excellent and thorough reviews are these:

Maeda, Patrick. Stanford University, "Zernike Polynomials and Their Use in Describing the Wavefront Aberrations of the Human Eye." This article is from a course, covering many mathematical details. The web site is http://scien.stanford.edu/class/psych221/projects/03/pmaeda/index.html
       and
Salmon, Thomas, "A Primer on Using Wavefront Analysis for Refractive Surgery and Other Ophthalmic Applications," likewise from a course, appears at http://www.opt.pacificu.edu/ce/catalog/10260-RS/WavefrontSalmon.html

---

[13] Available in summary form at the University of Georgia Libraries website, based on *The Chicago Manual of Style*, 15ed. (2003): http://libs.uga.edu/ref/chicago.html.

CLINICAL REFERENCES on the FOURIER SYSTEM

As mentioned, most web sites on Fourier are highly technical. Comparatively few clinically oriented articles on Fourier systems are available, but here are some helpful ones.

Ambrosio, Renato. "The Therapeutic Surface Ablation to Improve Vision Quality." 10th ESCRS Winter Refractive Surgery Meeting. Monte Carlo, *Grimaldi Forum*, Monaco (Feb. 2006): 10-12.

Chernyak, Dimitri. "Why Visx Switched to Fourier." *Cataract and Refractive Surgery* (Interview by A. Fagan, Senior Editor) (Jan. 2005): 55-58.

Holladay, Jack T. "Differences between Zernike, Fourier Have Limited Significance for Clinicians." *Ocular Surgery News* (11/1/2005) available at http://www.osnsupersite.com/default.asp?ID=11573.

Stevens, Julian. "Fourier Algorithms in Clinical Practice: The world's first case studies." *XXII Congress of the ESCRS*, Paris (2004): 15-22 Sept.

Vukich, John A. and Alio, Jorge L., chairs. "International Refractive Surgery: Science and Practice." *Refractive Surgery* (10/22/2004). A CD-ROM set is available.

Vukich, John A. "A. Fourier Algorithms for Driving Wavefront Ablations." *XXIII Congress of the ESCRS*, Paris (Sept. 2004): 15-22.

GENERAL REFERENCES

The most prolific authors, particularly on Zernike systems, are Thibos, Salmon and Liang. Many of their articles are published in the optometric journals.

Atchison D.A., Scott D.R. and Cox M.J. "Mathematical Treatment of Ocular Aberrations: a User's Guide." *Vision Science and Its Applications* 35 (2000): 110-30.

Campbell C.E. "A new method for describing the aberrations of the eye using Zemike polynomials." *Optom Vis Sci* (2003): 79-83.

Hersh P.E., Fry K. and Blaker W. "Spherical aberration after laser in site keratomileusis and photorefractive keratectomy; clinical results and theoretical models of etiology." *J Refract Surg* 29 (2003): 2096-2104.

Liang L., Grimm B., Goelz S. and Bille I. "Objective Measurement of Wave Aberrations of the Human Eye wih the use of a Hartmann-Shack Wave-front Sensor." *J. Opt. Soc. Am. A* Vol. 11, No.7 (1994): 1949-1957.

Liang J.W. "Aberration and Retinal Image Quality of the Normal Human Eye." *J Opt. Soc. Am. A* Vol. 14, No. 11 (1997): 2873-2883.

Liang J.W. and Miller D.T. "Supernormal vision and high-resolution retinal imaging through adaptive optics." *J Opt Soc Am. A* Vol. 14, No. 11 (1997): 2884-92.

MacRae S.M., Krueger R.R. and Applegate R.A. *Customized Corneal Ablation - The Quest for SuperVision.* Thorofare, NJ: SLACK, Inc., 2001.

Miller D.T. "Retinal Imaging and Vision at the Frontiers of Adaptive Optics." *Physics Today* 53 (2000): 31-36.

Platt Band Shack R. "History and Principles of Shack-Hartmann Waveftont Sensing." *J Ref Surg.* 17 (2001): 573-577.

Salmon T.O. "A Primer on Using Wavefront Analysis for Refractive Surgery and Other Ophthalmic Applications." Pacific University. http://www.opt.pacificu.edu/ce/catalogl/l0260-RS/WavefrontSalmon...

Salmon T.O. and West R.W. *Optical Wavefront Sensing of the Human Eye.* In: Pandalai S, ed. Recent Research in Optics, Fort, Trivandrum, India: Research Signpost (2002): 183-214.

Salmon T.O. and West R.W. "Measurement of Refractive Errors in Young Myopes Using the COAS Shack-Hartmann Aberrometer." *Optom Vis Sci* 80 (2003): 6-14.

Shiode Y. et al. "Method of Zernike Coefficients Extraction for Optical Aberration Measurement." www.usa.canon.com/html/industrial_semicondeq/pdfs/Method%20of%20Zernike.pdf

Thibos L.N. "Wavefront Data Reporting and Terminology." Form an article presented at the *Second International Wavefront Congress* in Monterey, CA. (2002): http://www.slackinc.com/eye/jrs/vol175/thibos.pdf

Thibos L.N. "Proposal for a VSIA taskforce on methods and standards for reporting aberration characteristics of eyes." Presented at the OSA topical meeting, Vision Science and Its Applications. Santa Fe: NM, Feb 21, 1999.

Thibos L.N. "The New Visual Optics." *Optom Vis Sci* 74 (1997): 465-466. http://research.opt.indiana.edu/Library/WavefrontReporting/

Thibos L.N, Applegate R.A., Schwiegerling J.T. and Webb R. "Standards for Reporting the Optical Aberrations of Eyes. OSA Trends in Optics and Photonics." *Vision science and its applications.* Vol 35, Vasudevan Lakshminarayanan, ed. Optical Society of America, Washington, DC (2000): 232-244.

Thibos L.N, Applegate R.A. and Marcos S. "Aberrometry: The Past, Present and Future of Optometry." *Optom Vis Sci.* 80 (2003): 1-2.

Thibos L.N. and Hong X. "Clinical Applications of the Shack-Hartmann Aberrometer." *Optom Vis Sci.*76 (1999): 817-825.

Thibos L.N., Cheng X. and Bradley A. "Design Principles and Limitations of Wavefront-guided Contact Lenses." Indiana University. http://research.opt.indiana.edu/library/waveGuidedLens/waveGuidedLens.html

Tolstoba N.D. "The Precision Testing Technique Development and the Investigation of Quality of the Main BTA Mirror Reflection Surface." http://aco.ifmo.ru/~nadinet

Yoon G.Y. and Williams D.R. "Visual performance after correcting the monochromatic and chromatic aberrations of the eye." *J Opt Soc Am A* 19 (2002): 266-275.

Wang J.Y, Silva D.E. "Wave-Front Interpretation with Zernike Polynomials." *Appl. Opt.* 19 (1980): 1510-1518.

Wyant J.C. University of Arizona "Zernike Polynomials." http://wyant.opt-sci.arizona.edu/zernikes/zernikes.htm

Zavyalove L.V. et al. "Automated Aberration Extraction Using Phase Wheel Targets." www.microe.rit.edu/research/lithography/research/aberrationmetro/ML5754188_zavyalova.pdf

Zavyalove L.V. et al. "Practical approach to full-field wavefront aberration measurement using phase wheel Targets." www.microe.rit.edu/research/lithography/research/aberrationmetro/6154-35-Zavyalova.pdf

AUTHOR'S PUBLICATIONS

All by Jagerman L.S. or Jagerman L.S. et al. None apply to Zernike or Fourier mathematics except "The Mathematics of Relativity for the Rest of Us."

"Ophthalmological Observations on Mesoridozine." *Am. J. Ophthal.* 69 (1970): 143-146

"Understanding Magnification in Ophthalmology: A Manual." Rochester, Minnesota: Amer. Acad. of Ophthal. and Otolaryng, 1970.

"Visual Acuity Measured with Easy and Difficult Optotypes in Normal and Amblyopic Eyes." *J. Ped. Ophthal.* 7 (1970): 49-54,

"Surgical Anatomy of the Orbital Floor." *Annals Ophthal.*, II (1970): 408-412.

"Appearance and Spontaneous Resolution of a Radiologic Sign of Orbital Floor Fracture." *J. Ped. Ophthal.*, 7 (1970): 171-173.

"Hering's Law Applied to the Near Reflex." *Am. J. Ophthal.* 70 (1970): 579-582.

"Safety Lenses in the Armed Forces." *Guild Guide* XXI, No. 4 (1970): 18-20.

"Studies in Refraction: The Precision of Retinoscopy." *Arch. Ophthal.* 84 (1970): 49-61

"Effects of Air Travel on Contact Lens Wearers." *Am. J. Ophthal.* 75, 3 (1973): 14-20.

"The Wearing of Hydrophilic Contact Lenses Aboard Commercial Jet Aircraft." *Aviation, Space and Environmental Medicine.* March (1982): 235-238.

"The Mathematics of Relativity for the Rest of Us." Victoria, Canada: Trafford Publishing, 2001.

96

INDEX

The numbers refer to *paragraph numbers* (not pages). The **bold numbers** refer to main occurrences.

Printed in the United States
By Bookmasters

Printed in the United States
By Bookmasters